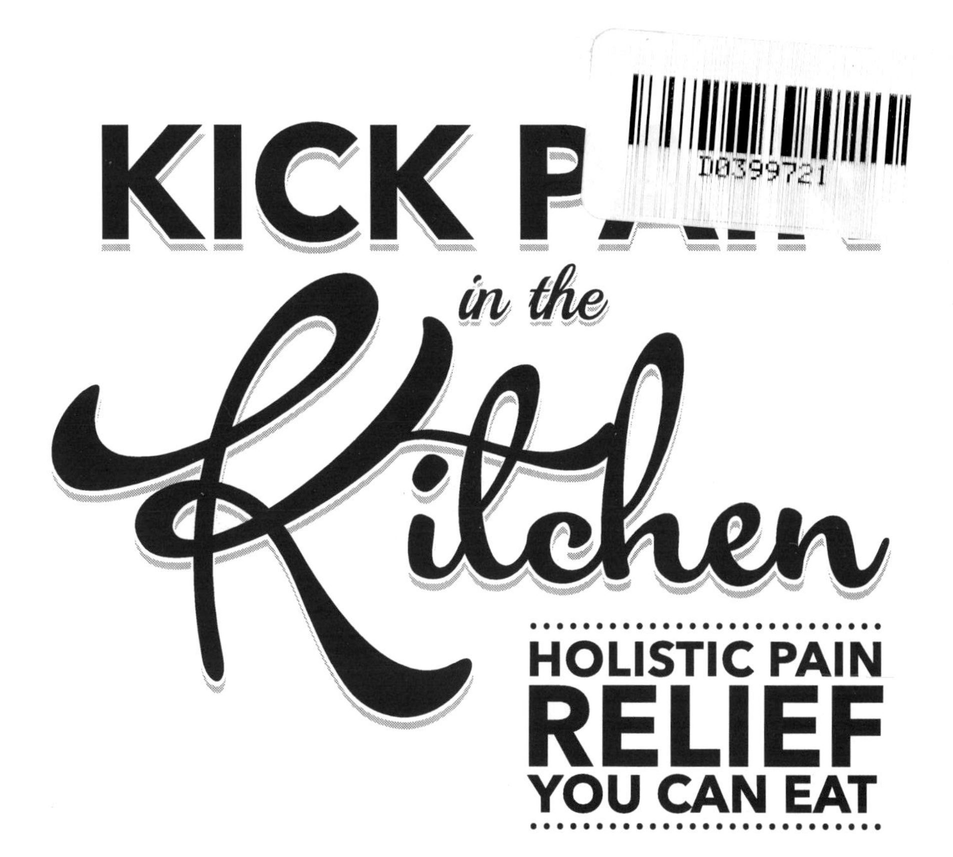

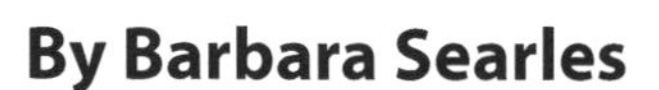

By Barbara Searles

Board-Certified Massage Therapist
&
Holistic Health Coach

Founder, ConfidentWellness.com

Printed in the United States of America

ISBN Paperback: 978-09906710-0-8
ISBN Digital: 978-0-9906710-1-5
Library of Congress Control Number: 2014918016

Printed by CreateSpace, An Amazon.com Company

Bodyworks Integrative Health, LLC
221B Rohrerstown Road
Lancaster, PA 17603

Editor: Author Connections, LLC, authorconnections.com
Cover design: Randall Graffa
Interior design: Cris Graffa
Author photo: Jeremy Madea, jeremymadea.com

www.kickpaininthekitchen.com

Visit the author's website at www.barbarasearles.com

First printing

For my clients, who each inspire and teach me every day.

For my dear friend, Jennifer, who gives tremendous love to the world while living gracefully with pain and chronic illness.

"Health doesn't happen in our doctor's office.
Health happens in our kitchen."

Mark Hyman, M.D.

Disclaimer

This book is a practical reference tool with information designed to assist readers who want to plan a holistic pain relief program. It is always best and strongly recommended to consult a medical doctor when making changes to your diet and/or lifestyle, so you can develop and execute a strategy that is truly best for your individual health, circumstance, and condition.

The materials and content contained in this book are for general health information only, and are not intended to be a substitute for professional medical advice, diagnosis or treatment.

Users of this book should not rely exclusively on information provided here for their own health needs. All specific medical questions should be presented to a professional health care provider.

The author makes no warranties or representations, express or implied, as to the accuracy or completeness, timeliness or usefulness of any opinions, advice, services, or other information contained or referenced in this book.

The information featured here is based exclusively on my personal experience as a business owner, a health coach, and a food lover living with pain.

Disclaimer of Health Related Services

The author encourages every reader to visit and consult proper healthcare professionals. The author is not acting in the capacity of a doctor, licensed dietician-nutritionist, psychologist, or other licensed or registered health professional. The author is not providing health care, medical, or nutrition therapy services, and shall not diagnose, treat or cure in any manner whatsoever any disease, condition, or other physical or mental ailment of the human body.

The ideas worded and presented here are 100% original, my own, and not intended to be medical advice, endorsements, or recommendations. I do hope that by sharing what I have learned on my own journey to managing pain, and how much I have been able to improve my lifestyle through changes in the kitchen, that it may help shed light on some new ideas for you to consider with proper medical guidance.

Table of Contents

Introduction 11

Part One: Changing the Foods We Eat for Holistic Pain Relief 13

Is This Book for You? 14

The Price of Pain 19

My Story 23

The Connection Between Inflammation and Pain 30

What's the Connection Between Gluten and Pain? 39

"Great-Grandmother Foods" 54

Dairy Products and Holistic Pain Relief 66

Hydrate or Die 70

Supplements 74

Part Two: Integrating Changes into Your Life 75

Putting Suggestions Into Action 76

Grocery Store 79

Breakfast 83

Lunch 87

Snacks 91

Dinner 96

Dessert 102

Events Away From Home 108

Making Pain-Relieving Food Choices When You Travel 113

Rethinking Your Kitchen 116

Part Three: The Human Aspects of Holistic Pain Relief 121

Other People 122

- Talking to Loved Ones (Especially Partners) About Going Gluten Free 122
- Connecting With Others Helps Minimize Pain 123
- But You Don't Look Sick 125

People Who Sabotage 126
Self-Care 128
How You Sleep is How You Do Everything 128
7 Tips for a Better Massage When You Live with Chronic Pain 130
Myofascial Release: A Different Kind of Bodywork 132
Integrating Movement Into Your Day 134
Would You Run a Mile in a Pool? 136
Negativity Detox 138
Mindset and Holistic Pain Relief 139

Part Four: Are You Ready for a Fresh Start? 143

Afterword 147

Acknowledgements 149

About the Author 151

Introduction

Barely six months ago, I was spending most of my days lying in my cool, dark bedroom reading novels. I'd get up and go to work when I could, seeing clients in my massage therapy and holistic pain relief coaching practice; but I often found myself all set for work, only to call the day's appointments and tell them I was too dizzy to stand up, much less give multiple massages over several hours. As long as I was stretched out on my bed with my head and neck completely supported, I was fine. Upright movement in any fashion was dicey; one moment it might be easy, and at other times simply standing still felt like standing on a boat in a hurricane.

On the days that I was able to work, my husband, Cris would take me to the office because I couldn't hear the traffic around me to drive safely. This hearing loss also made it dishearteningly difficult to communicate with clients, not to mention family and friends. Social activities were a combination of worrying what level of hearing I'd have that day, and wondering if we'd have to cancel at the last minute because I was too dizzy.

Cris and I were at the point of discussing the possibility of closing my business, applying for disability, and wondering what I'd be able to do with my life. Despite many appointments and consultations, I still had no idea what was causing the symptoms.

During these conversations, I sometimes found myself thinking of Toni Bernhard, the author of How to Be Sick, which I'd read a few months earlier. She left her career and became an author after finding herself ill and bed-bound with a mysterious ailment. I wondered if that would be my only option for communicating with clients, friends, and the world.

Fast-forward six months. I'm back on my feet and in my normal work, exercise, family, and social routine again. The diagnosis was made; treatment planned and carried out. I am well! I am living! I'll share more of the story as we go, and also the story of another important diagnosis and recovery. My gratitude to everyone who's supported me during this time is overflowing.

My professional training and personal experiences have been the foundation to a holistic pain relief process that I have developed for myself and for my clients. I love educating and encouraging people as they progress from living with debilitating daily pain to joyful freedom and pain relief. Now I want you to have that opportunity as well!

I know you're busy, and yet if you picked up this book it most likely means that you yourself or someone you love is living with chronic pain. I have been where you are, and I truly believe that reading this book can change your life, because the information here has changed mine. I've trimmed it down so you can finish this in one sitting. If the tips and instructions packed into this little book are a bit overwhelming, send me an email and I'll do my best to help. That is a promise.

Part One

Changing the Foods We Eat for Holistic Pain Relief

Is This Book for You?

According to one statistic, 116 million Americans have experienced chronic pain. If you're one of these struggling, suffering people, then this book is for you.

When I was in my 20s I remember someone saying you had to be "old" to talk with friends about one ailment or another, but as I got older myself I learned that chronic pain is actually common among people of all ages and lifestyles. Although sometimes I don't want a new friend to know I've experienced pain-related limitations, I'm often surprised at how quickly the topic surfaces when we share similar challenges. And since living with pain can be tremendously isolating, sometimes it helps to know we're not alone.

Let me say that again—you are *not* alone! This book shares my own story as well as stories from friends and clients. My hope is that reading this will help you feel a part of a welcoming and supportive community of people like yourself, searching for holistic pain relief.

The purpose of introducing my holistic pain relief process to you is to empower you in your own treatment of chronic pain. Living with chronic pain can make you feel like everyone is telling you what to do—doctors, physical therapists, even your mother-in-law! Taking control of your food and lifestyle choices and using them to create a holistic pain relief program can help you minimize pain and gain tremendous energy.

I cannot stress enough that these ideas and tips are not intended for use without proper medical guidance. Every individual is different and your personal needs and/or risks are not for me to address. I encourage you to discuss these options with your family, healthcare professionals, and physicians. The recommendations and instructions in this book integrate with all different kinds of pain relief treatment plans. My belief and experience is that making changes in your eating habits will *enhance* your existing options. Whether you can replace traditional methods or not is entirely up to you and your primary health care provider.

Who You Are:
Sometimes you feel like no one quite understands what it's like to live with chronic pain. It impacts every aspect of your life, keeping you from feeling positive and hopeful. You'd be willing to try just about anything to make progress or stop losing ground to pain. You might feel comfortable with either or both medical and holistic solutions, but don't know where to start.

What Your Issues Tend to Be:
Some days you don't have the energy to dive into life the way you'd like to. Pain levels slow you down and often take priority over the rest of your life. Pain keeps you from accomplishing tasks as quickly as you used to—things that were easy to accomplish in years past take a lot more time and effort now.

You lose sleep over the future because you can't be sure how pain will impact your life. Stress and worry make it hard to think positively about your body and overall situation.
You wish someone would explain not only the traditional options you have, but also the science and logic behind holistic solutions.

What You Need:
Lots of people approach you with unproven ideas and/or products to sell—you'd rather have straightforward solutions that don't cost a fortune and don't demand a lot of extra time. You need a set of realistic, simple tools that you can put in practice to minimize your pain and maximize your energy.

You may also feel like one of these stories describes you:

Recently diagnosed
Your mind is reeling from all the extra information you need to process. The doctors gave you some medication, and when you read the pharmacy insert, the side effects are pretty scary. In the middle of all this—you just plain hurt. It's exhausting, trying to learn what makes sense and trying to decide what to do next or where to begin.

Frustrated with the traditional approach
You've experienced the reality of the traditional approach to chronic pain for a year or more. You may be taking a few medications, and you may be coping with some nasty side effects. Juggling treatment plans is wearing you out. Sometimes it feels like a second job, managing your pain and/or illness; and you're thinking there must be another way to get relief—a natural regimen focused on small daily changes with fewer side effects and better results. But researching holistic options is confusing, and it would be an enormous help to have someone more experienced act as your filter, to distill all the data down to a simple, easy to follow process.

Exploring all the options
You're using all the medical and holistic methods you know of to feel energetic and pain-free, but it's not working. You've already tried what feels like a half million recommended remedies to find solutions to the pain that plagues you, but so much of the information available is conflicting, confusing,

and overwhelming. You need to fully comprehend the variety of solutions for chronic pain, to see which routine is best for you. How incredible would it be to have someone help you make sense of it all?

Are You Ready to Participate in Your Healing?

No matter what your diagnosis or situation might be, if you are ready to participate in the process of being healed, this book is for you. Even if you aren't yourself living with chronic pain per se, we all have aches and pains as we age, and many of the tips and recipes in this book can help you feel your best and live your best life, longer. If you are in fact the reader this book is written for, a patient living with chronic pain, don't give up hope! With continued research, study, trial and error, you might eventually find health care or allied health professionals who are able to fix the pain you're living with. If you are that fortunate at some point down the road, all the power to you! This book, however, is intended to help right now, today, before any miracle comes knocking on your door. You don't need to passively wait and hope for relief, because with a little guidance and support you can take back some control, regain some independence, and relieve some of your own pain by tapping into the innate strength and ability you *already* have.

I believe it is up to each of us to work through our challenges toward the progress we need. That doesn't mean it's easy or that we don't need help. As you will see in upcoming chapters, I learned to view my own illness and chronic pain management as a team effort. I enlisted other team members (medical and holistic), but it was up to me to be in charge. Even if I found an amazing coach who had a fantastic approach that made me feel like I was winning my health back, I couldn't let that coach run *all* the plays. I had to get in there and make decisions, make changes that were the best fit for my family and lifestyle, and be willing to learn new things.

I've found that taking a team approach wins the game, and I encourage you to be the captain of your own team. I invite you to join with me as your holistic pain relief coach. I can help you develop a plan that is crafted for you and your team. This "healing team" concept started for me when massage therapy clients came in thanking me for "fixing" or "healing" them. Honestly, it makes me uncomfortable to be the only reason someone feels better—I prefer when clients take an active part in the process, so I always tell clients that this is a team effort. In the case of massage therapy, the team has three members: me as therapist, the client as a willing mental and emotional participant, and the client's body as the important third. It may seem strange to perceive your body as separate from your mind, because of course they're connected and part of the whole you, but sometimes when we live with chronic pain it feels like our *body is separate,* since it's doing things we'd rather it didn't—like hurt. I encourage you to acknowledge and be easy with those feelings. Invite your body to join your team, and face the challenge together.

It's okay if you'd prefer to give the responsibility for healing your chronic pain to someone else. Sometimes we get so beaten down by the experience of living with chronic pain that we have no energy left to do another thing. Believe me, I hear you. But you picked up this book, so the idea of taking an active role in the process must intrigue you. Go ahead, read a little further. You may find that this approach is much easier than you think.

I lived with chronic pain for a long time. I've been in your shoes. If you find at least one or two ideas here that you can implement to better manage your pain, my mission with this little book will be accomplished. Just one or two changes can gain you the energy you need to resume a more active and comfortable role in your daily life. Imagine that!

The Price of Pain

How long have you been living with chronic pain? Medically, pain is considered chronic when it has continued for six months or more. That sounds so dispassionate and distant, doesn't it? As if six months isn't such a big deal. I know and you know that by the time chronic pain has lingered for months instead of weeks, it's already wreaked havoc on our lives. It changes who we are and how we relate to the world around us.

I lived with mild chronic back pain in my 20s, moderate chronic pain in my back and knees in my 30s, and the serious, chronic pain of multiple involved joints and major fatigue in my early 40s. By the time I reached my mid 40s, I had lived with chronic pain for so long that I honestly had no idea this wasn't how everyone felt!

I tell you this not to make you feel sorry for me, because during this time I actually lived a full and satisfying life. I had a career I loved, enriching family and love relationships, and plenty of life challenges, too. I found a way to integrate chronic pain into my life, never realizing that my co-workers might not be thinking about pain in the midst of pursuing their career goals.

It is important to acknowledge here that I *understand* how it feels to live with pain. I've been there, too. I realize how essential it is to feel personal connections, because living with pain can make us feel terribly isolated from the other people in our lives (especially when they can't relate to our suffering, why we cancel plans, why we are always tired).

Have you ever thought about the cost of living with chronic pain? Maybe wished that some of that cost could be relieved? I believe we each have our own story of pain. Connected to that story is a set of costs individual to us—but similar to other people living with chronic pain.

As a holistic pain relief coach and massage therapist, I often talk with clients about the price of living with chronic pain. What are the costs you can think of right away? And remember, your time has a value associated with it. Is there an hourly rate you (or your employer) charge for your time? Our time is valuable—what would you do with yours if you weren't using it to manage your chronic pain?

Here are some ways to quantify the price of pain:

- Time and money to see physicians and specialists (often more than one)
- Time and money for managing medications (even if you've got a pharmacy that delivers)
- Time and money for managing non-invasive or invasive treatment plans like physical therapy, cortisone shots, and/or surgery
- Hours and nights of sleep lost (plus new mattresses and pillows bought just in case the pain was their fault!)
- Productivity at work lost (and the emotional price of worrying about job security)
- Counseling to manage the emotional impact on you and the people around you
- Income lost due to short-term or long-term disability

- Paid time off used (*if* you have that job benefit)
- Time with family lost or not enjoyed as you'd like
- Time with friends lost or not enjoyed as you'd like
- Costs of non-medical help like housekeeping, lawn mowing, etc.
- Costs of integrative help not always covered by medical insurance like acupuncture, massage, chiropractic, etc.

Take a moment right now, and think about what you'd add to this list from your own experience. Now take a deep breath in and let it all out. You wouldn't be here with me now if you weren't wishing for some answers. I'm here to tell you there are small changes you can make to start gaining holistic pain relief. That's what this book is about! We'll cover lots of small changes—you choose how to implement them in your life so it's realistic and manageable.

At the height of my chronic pain (now a few years ago), I felt like managing my situation was a full-time job in itself. Plus, as an entrepreneur, I didn't have paid sick time or vacation time to help defray the costs of all the lost sleep and working hours. At the time, there was also a long-term cost because I was considered uninsurable for private health insurance, and so I was paying cash out of pocket for all medical appointments and prescriptions. I was exhausted and *unbearably* stressed; plus, don't forget, hurting!

Wouldn't you agree that these are pretty strong motivators to finding solutions and making changes? Well, that's exactly how I felt and why I started looking at holistic pain relief solutions for my own situation.

First I worked with my own choices—improving the nutrition in the food I ate and removing inflammatory foods, as well as enhancing the holistic ways I nurtured myself. As my health coaching and massage clients began to notice that my own pain was improving, they asked me to help them, too.

Together with my clients, I started to develop a process that offers holistic pain relief by focusing on these essential elements:

1. Increase High Quality Food and Maximize Nutrition
2. Understand Inflammatory Foods and Bio-Individuality
3. Eliminate Your Inflammatory Foods
4. Enhance Self-Care Practices
5. Network Within Your Community and Expand Connections with Others

Sound good?

Keep reading!

In this book, I'll be sharing these elements with you and giving you the tools you need to Kick Pain in the Kitchen!

My Story

How it Started: Inflammatory Autoimmune Arthritis

In 2002, when I started transitioning from my corporate career to a solo entrepreneurial massage therapy practice, I began to understand that caring for my hands and my body was essential to my business success. Massage therapists depend on their own bodies to help make their clients' bodies feel better. Our massage therapy instructors taught us hand-strengthening exercises. We learned the benefits of an ice pack on our hands after a few massages. I also started receiving more regular massage for myself—about one for every ten I gave to others.

You can imagine what it felt like six years later when my hands, fingers and wrists started experiencing pain and swelling. It scared me because my hands are my tools—I can't do my job if they don't work properly! I started by trying to solve the pain and swelling on my own, using massage techniques. I asked the massage therapists who worked on me to spend extra time on my hands. I rubbed my own hands and fingers at the end of most workdays, and used a lot more ice packs than I had the previous year, but the swelling and pain continued. Since my typical solutions didn't help, after a few months I progressed to getting medical advice and blood tests. Eventually, three days before my 45th birthday, I was officially diagnosed with inflammatory autoimmune (often called rheumatoid) arthritis.

Not long after this, I was entirely freaked out because even the anti-inflammatory medications weren't making any difference. My brain works overtime, especially when I need to solve problems, and this chronic, inflammatory pain situation was sending my brain to one place over and over again: Would I still be able to be a massage therapist and run my thriving solo practice? My business was hectic—I had a full schedule giving about 25 massages each week. I was terrified of losing it all to the effects of a disease.

In a critical step towards my wellness, I found a new rheumatologist who was a better fit for my personality. I will never forget that moment during our first hour-long appointment when I asked him, "Does having inflammatory autoimmune arthritis mean I'll need to give up this profession and business that I love?" He looked back at me and said with great sincerity, "Absolutely not—that would mean giving up something that means too much to you and makes you who you are." What a priceless gift of stress relief that one statement was!

Eighteen months later, my rheumatologist declared my arthritis in remission. He's not used to patients coming in with high heels on, but I now do exactly that. He's not used to people who thrive with the smallest medicine doses possible, but I am; and we're both thrilled that my massage therapy practice isn't limited because of *my* pain.

My rheumatologist supports my holistic approach because he sees results. He says, "Whatever you're doing is working, so keep doing it!"

So, what is it that I do to thrive with inflammatory autoimmune arthritis?

Well, I do take medication—the lowest doses possible and no anti-inflammatories, prednisone, or biologics. I also eat primarily whole, non-processed, home-cooked foods. I initially minimized wheat and now am completely gluten free. I do yoga or water exercise at least 2–3 days each week, and I make sure to get plenty of sleep and relaxation time.

I'm purposefully intentional about how I describe arthritis and autoimmunity in my body. It may sound hokey, but to me it's important that I never refer to the autoimmune aspects of this disease as my body attacking itself. These are common words in the medical community, but they make me feel as if my diagnosis is a losing battle. That isn't the way I want to approach something I plan to overcome!

Inflammatory autoimmune arthritis has brought me to a new place in my career and entrepreneurial life. During the diagnosis process, I decided to pursue my long-standing interest in wellness and nutrition by getting certified as a Holistic Health Coach. Naturally, I also wanted to use that education to have more resources and information at my own disposal. Health coaching people who, like me, have chronic pain, is now my mission.

Next Came Migraine

After a few years of working with clients to help them reduce their pain and inflammation, I had an incredibly hectic life as owner of two businesses. I'm also a wife, mother, daughter, and grandmother. Plus, I'm continually trying to make time to take care of my own health.

Worn down and not caring properly for myself, I caught a cold, which developed into a sinus infection. Just as I started to feel better, the symptoms returned. The highs and lows of alternately feeling better and worse continued for several weeks. During some of the tough intervals, I had vertigo and quite a bit of disequilibrium. Disequilibrium is when you feel like you're on a boat—but you're not! These experiences combined can be very disconcerting. Then I started to lose hearing in my right ear, including a distortion of low-frequency sounds, like men's voices.

My bad days started to outnumber the good. Things were going from challenging to debilitating, and despite many appointments and tests, I still didn't have any answers. Some medications (like prednisone) worked for a time, but didn't solve the problem and had scary possible side effects. I was way too sick to seek, discover and confirm more effective holistic treatment methods, except for getting lots of rest. After visiting doctors, chiropractors, clinical nutritionists, and acupuncturists, no one could tell me what was wrong or how to fix it.

This is when Cris started driving me to and from my massage office, because I simply couldn't do it. Many times I had to cancel client appointments at the last minute because I couldn't stand up, much less give a massage. We were researching the possibility of me going on government disability. I spent almost all day in bed, reading. During this time I read 20+ books in eight weeks.

Along my journey I was eventually referred to a specialist who spent about twenty minutes talking with me about my symptoms. We also talked about the progression of symptoms over not only the several months before our appointment, but many years prior. When he told me that all of my symptoms were caused by migraine activity, I could have fallen out of my chair, because I only get the occasional tension headache! In all the years I've been doing bodywork and coaching, I've treated loads of people living with migraine, and every time I've been grateful that I didn't live with that kind of pain.

Although I had some intuition that food was part of the problem and/or solution, never in a million years did I expect a doctor to tell me that I needed an elimination diet. Most physicians have limited training in nutrition, and in my holistic healing work I have a LOT of training in nutrition. I never anticipated being told that dietary changes were the necessary path for me. This was a big lesson to learn—that sometimes there's a LOT more to a condition than you realize. Migraine is simply inflammation of the blood vessels in your head and neck, sometimes shoulders; and because of their location near the brain and nervous system, that inflammation can affect many different bodily functions.

I was far from alone. Over 37 million people in the U.S. alone cope with migraines. It is one of the most common pain-related conditions keeping people from participating fully in their lives.

Migraine symptoms affect many systems of your body—not only your head. And many things, including what we eat and drink, can trigger migraine activity. Since we have control over what we swallow, a migraine trigger elimination diet was the first step for me.

I thought going gluten-free for autoimmune inflammatory arthritis was tough, but the elimination diet was tougher. On the up side, I experienced *huge* symptom relief within just 2–3 weeks.

Your Takeaway:

- You're not alone in facing pain challenges and the need to learn how to find answers.
- Food and nutrition are intimately connected to wellness.
- Persist in looking for solutions that will help you. Pace yourself, but don't give up.
- Asking for help is okay.

All of my chronic pain experiences have been (and continue to be) life changing. If in some small way my story brings you hope and motivation to take action for yourself, then I've done what I set out to do.

Massage Therapist

In my practice I've given thousands of massages in the last eleven years. Some clients I see once, while others I see once a week for years at a time. It all depends on what helps them feel pain relief. It's all bio-individual.

When I was in massage therapy school I thought to myself, *I'm so stressed in my corporate career that I just want non-stressful clients—people who mostly want to focus on how to relax.* Well, the truth is that relief from corporate work wasn't my only interest. As clients with more complex pain-related situations came to see me, for the first time I saw a purpose for my own chronic pain, because it gives me tremendous perspective as a therapist and coach. When someone needs my help relieving pain, I am able to look them in the eye and genuinely say, "I know how you feel."

As time passed I realized that *most* of my clients had some level of chronic pain; it made perfect sense for this to be my specialty, and I love the challenge of helping people feel better and return to their lives. It's my calling now, far more than a job or business career.

Holistic Health Coach

In my twenties, I lost about forty pounds using Weight Watchers. This sparked a flame inside me, a passion for nutrition information. I always gravitate to those articles in magazines. My clients and I often talk about nutrition trends, issues or questions. About a month after graduating massage school, I received a catalog from the Institute for Integrative Nutrition (IIN). I devoured the information, especially the idea of bio-individuality, and felt inspired that such a school exists, but first I needed to focus on the transition from corporate career to independent massage therapist. One thing at a time.

After a while, I met an IIN-trained health coach and worked with her for a six-month course. We've remained close friends ever since, and I'm incredibly blessed to have been through her program.

When the diagnosis of inflammatory autoimmune arthritis came to me, I knew it was time to become a holistic health coach. As a student and graduate of IIN I've studied over 100 different nutritional theories directly from the world's leading experts. Integrating these varied approaches to benefit myself and my clients has been an amazing journey, both personally and professionally.

Holistic Pain Relief Coach

I now use the term Holistic Pain Relief Coach to describe what I do, because it combines all the chapters of my background and experience. What I believe matters most is not the knowledge I've gained in itself, but the ability to translate what I know into practical solutions for my clients, so they can each find their own path toward pain relief.

As a person living with chronic pain I often wished for a mentor to help me navigate my options, and that's the type of mentoring I provide to my clients; information from someone who's been in their shoes and come out the other side with new energy, hope, and perspective.

The Connection Between Inflammation and Pain

Why talk about inflammation?

It's simple: Too much inflammation is a huge factor in chronic pain. Plus, finding ways to control and limit inflammation is a key strategy in holistic pain relief.

First, what do I mean by systemic inflammation?

Systemic inflammation is throughout your entire body—throughout all the systems. It's not that localized inflammation you see when you fall and your knee swells. Systemic inflammation generally develops over time, can become chronic, and is the result of a variety of different factors.

Fundamentally, inflammation is your body's natural protective response; but left unchecked, it can actually cause more inflammation, so understanding your bio-individual inflammatory process and getting it under control are essential steps in holistic pain relief.

Some chronic pain-related diseases and conditions include chronic peptic ulcers, autoimmune arthritis, chronic periodontitis, ulcerative colitis and Crohn's disease, acid reflux, and chronic sinusitis. These are only a few; there are many more. In some cases inflammation comes from sources other than disease. Such alternate sources are most likely lifestyle choices—the way you sleep or eat, for example. Some people may notice discomfort and pain before a disease has reached the stage of diagnosis. Noticing certain changes helps to address the inflammation before it takes over and gets out of control.

Here are some of the main factors in chronic, systemic inflammation:

1. Environmental factors: Toxins in our world are creating chronic inflammation in our bodies. You've probably heard about the huge variety of toxic ingredients in everything from cleaning products to cookware, furniture, and carpeting. Being aware of toxins as a frequent cause of inflammation and pain is the first step to making healthy changes. Food choices also can add to our toxic intake. Most processed foods (found in boxes and bags on supermarket shelves) have been made with genetically modified organisms (GMO) ingredients. This can mean that those foods have pesticides and other chemicals built right into their genetic structure.
2. Poor diet: Certain foods, especially sugar, refined flours, processed ingredients, and trans or saturated fats are a big factor in chronic pain because of their relationship to inflammation. Even choosing organic sugar (or a sugar-type product) can potentially feed the inflammation in your body! Later in this book we'll talk further about how to judge what types of foods are inflammatory or not. For now, just know that the more refined and processed a food is, the more likely it is to cause inflammation in your body.
3. Gut/digestive issues: Your gut (which is another way to say your intestinal tract) may not be a place you think about having inflammation. It may feel inflamed or bloated, it may not. The feeling of being 'out of balance' can come and go over time. Since your gut contains 60–70% of your

immune system, an inflamed gut can wreak major havoc throughout your whole body. This becomes more of an issue when the gut is out of balance for a long time—over years vs. only weeks or months. Many things can damage the gut's natural bacterial balance: antibiotics and other medicines, food allergies/intolerances, environmental and food toxins, and toxic buildup resulting from constipation. When your gut bacteria are out of balance it creates inflammation in the gut, which can also contribute to toxins leaking into the rest of your body.

4. Chronic stress: You probably know from your own experience that chronic stress (lasting at least 3 months) makes it hard to stay well. In 2013, a study[1] found that chronic stress actually changes our genes. It changes immune cells into 'fighter' cells before they enter the bloodstream, and this happens whether or not there's actually infection or trauma present for that immune cell to fight. Having these 'fighter' cells in our bloodstream then spreads inflammation throughout our bodies.

5. Poor sleep quality: Scientists at Emory University School of Medicine in Atlanta, Georgia found[2] that "Poor sleep quality, and short sleep durations are associated with higher levels of inflammation." One of the best ways for the body to heal and de-stress is to get a good night's sleep, but for many of us this kind of sleep is elusive, especially when you're experiencing pain. You get caught up in an intense TV show just before bed, and it's hard to wind down. You have a hard time shutting down the worries and stresses of the day. You fall asleep on the couch just after dinner and the evening nap makes it hard to sleep

[1] http://www.huffingtonpost.com/2013/11/07/chronic-stress-health-inflammation-genes_n_4226420.html

[2] http://www.medicalnewstoday.com/articles/207877.php

through the night. Are any of these familiar? As the book offers ways to address holistic pain relief, I'll cover ways to get better sleep each night, too.

6. Lack of exercise/sedentary lifestyle: It's no secret that exercise is critical to long-term wellness. Not a day goes by that I don't see fitness advice on TV, in a magazine, or on social media. But, when we're living with chronic pain, exercise sometimes seems like the most impossible thing. Later in this book we'll talk about ideas for integrating movement into each day. There are so many benefits to increasing movement and exercise in our lives. For example, when your skeletal muscles perform work, they actually produce and release anti-inflammatory substances into the blood. So staying still and not exercising is a big part of chronic, systemic inflammation, and getting moving (even just a little) will make you feel less pain.
7. Carrying extra weight: Studies[3] show that even a 5% weight loss can reduce inflammatory markers in blood tests. The good news is that if you make changes in some of the other items on this list, you will naturally give your body the opportunity to release weight. For example, better sleep and high quality food are both associated with weight loss. Small changes work together in our lives to make a big impact on pain levels.

Making all these changes at once may seem overwhelming, but as we get deeper into each idea, I'll teach you ways to make small changes in manageable steps. Since change can be stressful, and stress is a part of inflammation, it's best to get coaching and support when overhauling your lifestyle.

[3] http://www.medicalnewstoday.com/releases/244852.php

Let me say that again...*small* changes work together in our lives to make a *big* impact on our pain levels. Feeling better shouldn't be excruciating. My goal is to offer you ways to feel better that you can incorporate in your life *right now.*

Bio-individuality of inflammation

Bio-individuality simply means that not everyone's body responds in exactly the same way to the same food, exercise, or other habits. One person's solution or positive step, when applied to another person, can be less helpful or even destructive. Every body and its unique biology are individual. This means our reactions to lifestyle choices are uniquely our own. In the same vein, our reactions to certain foods are bio-individual—for example, how much any one food inflames your body.

I think about inflammation and pain as a puzzle. I wish it were a simple puzzle, the kind that toddlers play with; but unfortunately, for most of us it's a much more complicated and multi-layered mystery. We have to really tune in to our bodies to figure out which pieces to remove first and how everything shifts around.

Here's an example: Have you seen any of the images or articles about green drinks lately? For a while I was seeing these ideas and recipes everywhere, so I started to think it was a great idea for me. I found a recipe that included a green apple, kale, water, and half a lemon. And I *loved* it—so much that I was drinking this green drink every day. I made so much that I drank a big glass in the morning and another in the afternoon. And after about four weeks, I realized that my hands were swelling. I'm very mindful of my hands because I use them all day giving massage to clients—and they were uncomfortable.

I had to go back to the puzzle of my inflammation and pain to try to figure out what I'd shifted around recently. After some detective work, it seemed that the lemon in my green drink might be the problem. Best solution? Just stop the green drink completely. Within 48 hours my hands had returned to 100% normal, and that was enough proof for me. Even healthy options can work against you if ingested incorrectly or in the wrong doses. This is why it is so important to be aware of your own bio-individual needs and limitations.

This doesn't mean that I'll never use lemon again, and this recipe for green drinks could be great for you or someone else. From this experience, I learned that my body prefers I moderate my use of lemon. Half a lemon (including juice and pulp) every day is too much for me. But I do use it in other ways, as a flavoring in healthy sauces or squeezed on some fish. As you might imagine, I wasn't surprised when I saw lemon and citrus on the list of possible migraine triggers. That confirmed what my puzzle work had already taught me.

Bio-individuality sounds like a great concept—and it is. But here's a truth: sometimes it can be very difficult to figure out exactly what your body responds to (either positively or negatively) and why. When you are trying to determine your own bio-individual needs and tendencies, is the perfect time to engage the help of a health or holistic pain relief coach. Professionals like myself are trained to stand back and be objective about our clients' choices. We help you determine which inflammatory foods are giving you the most trouble, and more importantly, which *anti-inflammatory* choices will bring you the most relief. Coach and client experiment together, and collective knowledge makes the process work. It also can bring tremendous comfort and stress reduction to have an experienced guide remind you that you are not alone, and help you follow a structured path toward wellness, even if the start of that path includes some trial and error as you discover your bio-individual makeup. As stated earlier, stress reduction is a significant factor in pain/inflammation reduction and overall wellness, so a holistic health coach can both ease and foster your journey.

Fundamentals of an anti-inflammatory diet:
Inflammation is common today because our bodies are out of balance. Our bodies use nutrients from the food we eat as raw material to produce chemicals called prostaglandins. The major nutrients that our bodies use to create prostaglandins are omega-3 or omega-6 fatty acids. Omega-3 fatty acids produce an anti-inflammatory response in our bodies. Omega-6 fatty acids produce an inflammatory response. Our bodies need an equal amount of each to maintain a balanced inflammatory status. However, today's standard American diet provides up to 20 times more omega-6 fatty acid than omega-3. My goal is to help you identify food choices that will keep your body balanced in the positive, anti-inflammatory range.

What are significant sources of inflammatory omega-6 fatty acids?
Sweets, starches (especially grains), and highly processed foods are the main culprits. We consume more cereal grains (and the oils produced from them) than ever before.

In addition, the animals we eat are also consuming increased quantities of grains (primarily corn). Even fish are being corn-fed in farms that raise seafood to meet growing demands.

Does this mean I have to follow a highly restrictive diet?

No—it simply means you need to be aware of the balance of nutrients your body is receiving. You'll want to make nutritional choices that support your body's natural desire for a balanced equilibrium of anti- and pro-inflammatory responses.

Components of an anti-inflammatory diet:
Focus on meats, fish, eggs, and lots of fresh, leafy vegetables.

1. Low starch and other simple sugars: Insulin and high blood glucose are inflammatory. Consume starch only in small portions (½ banana or small sweet potato) and preferably in unprocessed forms. Aim for less than 30 grams in any meal—less is healthier.

2. No high fructose corn syrup: High fructose corn syrup (a fruit-derived sugar not bound to another type of sugar molecule like glucose) is inflammatory and contributes to cross-linking of collagen fibers, which means prematurely aged skin. These collagen fibers are also a big part of what make up our muscles, fascia, bones, ligaments, and tendons. When collagen is inflamed it can contribute to pain in any or all of these structures. However, know this: although high fructose corn syrup is inflammatory, it is not better to switch to artificial sweeteners! Artificial sweeteners are even more inflammatory than sucrose, which is table or white sugar.

3. High ratio of omega-3 to omega-6 fatty acids: Most vegetable oils (olive oil is the exception) are very high in omega-6 fats and inflammatory. These should be avoided. Omega-3 fats from fish oil cannot have their full anti-inflammatory impact in the presence of vegetable oils, so consider how you cook them. Omega-3 supplements are often needed to overcome existing inflammation. For maximum absorption, be sure to take with a meal when you also eat saturated fats.

4. No trans fats: All trans fats are inflammatory. Read ingredient lists and look for the words "hydrogenated" or "partially hydrogenated." Don't believe "no trans fats" claims without reading the ingredient list.

5. Probiotics and prebiotics: The bacteria in your gut are vitally important in reducing inflammation. Most of the bacteria in breast milk and also present in fermented products seem to be beneficial. A high-quality probiotic supplement can also be quite helpful.

6. Saturated fats are healthy; they reduce the oxidation of omega-3 fatty acids at local inflammation sites (e.g. fatty liver). Saturated fats should be a significant source of dietary calories to help balance you towards anti-inflammation. Vegetable oils (corn, soy, cottonseed, safflower) are rich in omega-6 fatty acids and are dangerously inflammatory. These polyunsaturated oils are less healthy than saturated fats. Olive oil is the healthiest choice.

7. Vegetable antioxidants: Vegetables and fruits along with coffee and dark chocolate supply powerful anti-inflammatory antioxidants.

5 What's the Connection Between Gluten and Pain?

Gluten is a major factor in our diets today, but what IS gluten, exactly? Even the word gluten, which is the Latin word for glue, gives us a clue about what it can do in our bodies.

Gluten is the combination of two parts of the wheat plant—gliadin and glutenin. These two ingredients join together with another starch and comprise 80% of the protein found in wheat. It makes wheat dough elastic and able to rise. It's also used in many imitation meat products to add protein—like imitation crab or the vegetarian protein called seitan.

Gluten is found in wheat, rye, barley, and in most commercially produced oats. Most of us get the majority of our gluten from wheat, so sometimes I'll use those two terms interchangeably here.

When I started to learn about how wheat has changed since the early 20th century, I was amazed. The entire history is pretty long and involved, so I'll summarize it briefly for you. Wheat was always planted with plenty of space between the rows, because that's what kept it from getting diseased. In the 1950s and 1960s, a "Green Revolution" began that changed the way wheat was grown[4]. Using chemical and genetic advancements, wheat was made resistant to drought, disease, and pests. All of this was done without regard to short or long term effects on the humans consuming it. Now, wheat can be grown much closer together and still not get diseased.

A dwarf version of wheat was also created, so that more actual wheat fruit grew at the top of each (now shorter) stalk. Then genetics were rearranged again, to allow for better "baking properties"—more consistent, fluffier results.

Maybe this all sounds pretty harmless, but note that there are no requirements to test any of these hybridizations or genetic modifications (GMO) on humans. Although the wheat industry was much happier with how much wheat they could produce in a square acre of land, people eating wheat had no idea how these engineered versions affect their bodies.

Then the wheat industry got even savvier, and started to genetically adjust wheat so that it actually makes people who eat it feel **addicted** to it! Works for the industry, right? They feed us a type of wheat that makes us all want more wheat. But, like any other addiction, there's always a dark side.

It makes me mad that someone (or some big industry) would hook an entire population on something without ever telling those people what could happen. And after a good deal of education on this topic, I am suspicious about whether wheat is actually as healthy as we're taught. It's bio-individual—wheat can be a big problem for some people, and a much smaller one or no problem at all for others.

[4] http://www.grainstorm.com/pages/rant

You may have heard about people who have major autoimmune reactions to gluten—they have what's called celiac disease. There is even some controversy about non-celiac gluten intolerance. This is a situation where someone doesn't test positive for celiac disease, but has significant sensitivities to gluten. For many people that sensitivity shows up as pain or inflammatory conditions.

A lot of study about gluten is going on at the National Institutes of Health (NIH) in the U.S. In fact, their online archive shows that studies have been published linking no less than 15 pain-related conditions to gluten consumption. Some of these include: restless leg syndrome, autoimmune arthritis, osteoarthritis, migraines, carpal tunnel syndrome, and more.

I know that when I was diagnosed with inflammatory autoimmune arthritis, people from many different parts of my life started mentioning gluten intolerance. I wasn't ready to listen because I LOVED my breads. I actually waited three years to eliminate gluten completely, because I needed to see the science before I'd make the effort to give up this yummy stuff. Not only did I see the studies, but I also read several books and articles from credible, trusted authors discussing the type of trigger that gluten can be for inflammation.

I read recently about one of the most direct connections between gluten and inflammation in a book called *Clean Gut*, by Alejandro Junger, M.D. Junger is not alone in saying that gluten is one of the major irritants to our gut—the intestinal tract. Ever had a big pizza and felt really bloated afterwards? Wondering how this connects to pain? The more upset and out of sorts your gut is, the more gas and undigested stuff it contains. It simply gets really full of...stuff... which pushes on your lower back from the inside. Don't forget—this part of our body is the front of our lower back; the lower back is right behind the gut. In fact, they are only inches from each other and, in a sense, completely connected. So doesn't it make sense that the 43% of U.S. workers reporting back pain might have some gluten and gut issues? How many millions of people is 43% of a work force? If this connection is true for even a quarter of that number, it's got to be seriously considered.

Information like this made me decide to give complete gluten elimination a try. I'd already been weaning myself over the course of three years, and the time had come.

Now, if you're not ready to go completely gluten-free, you may get some anti-inflammatory benefit from simply reducing your gluten intake. I say *may* get some relief, because each of us is different. This is an individual choice and you essentially have two ways to approach it. You can begin by first eliminating gluten in one meal every day (breakfast, for example). Or you can choose a short period of time like 3 weeks and try complete gluten elimination, to see if it makes a difference. We'll talk more about specific strategies in Part Two.

Identifying Gluten on Food Labels

My intention here is not to teach you all the details about going gluten-free. There are many books and web sites that cover this information thoroughly, and it's too big of a topic for this book. In fact, I've already written, "The Gluten-Free Detox Guide," which has loads of delicious and important details. You can find it at www.confidentwellness.com/gluten.

Eating gluten free (GF) for pain relief doesn't mean going into the "Gluten-Free" food aisle in the supermarket and simply trading your old crackers for GF crackers; or the old version of any type of processed food for a GF version of that same processed food. Processed food is most likely part of the problem with your chronic pain. Gluten-free processed food is not the solution!

When going gluten free, the best policy is to keep your focus on foods that don't have extensive labeling. The solution begins with whole, fresh foods. Go for lots of vegetables and fruits—plus proteins (sustainable meat or vegetarian choices), and naturally GF complex carbohydrates like sweet potatoes and quinoa. Making these types of changes can be incredibly satisfying—I promise!

Here are a few of the sneaky places you may not expect to see gluten—but it's in there.

- Beer
- Blue cheese
- Cereals
- Instant coffee
- Croutons
- Dairy substitutes
- Deli meats
- Gravy
- HVP (hydrolyzed vegetable protein)
- Imitation seafood
- Marinades
- Salad dressings
- Seasonings
- Soy sauce
- Emulsifiers
- Fillers
- Thickeners
- Modified food starch

- Malt
- Natural flavors

Even when you choose to eat primarily whole, naturally GF foods, there are times when you'll choose to eat foods with labels (even less processed foods will have some type of label). If your goal is to eat primarily or completely gluten free for pain relief, you want to learn to read labels on **everything**.

In terms of labels, products without gluten may say any of the following on the package:

- Gluten-free
- Without gluten
- Free of gluten
- No gluten

As of August 2014, U.S. standards state that products marked with any of these phrases can contain up to 20 parts per million (that's 0.002%) of gluten and still be labeled as Gluten-Free.

You can be quite comfortable with "Certified Gluten-Free" products. This specific label indicates that the product has met strict GF quality standards[5]. However, the best policy is always to read the entire ingredient list carefully.

Here's an extensive list[6] of ingredients containing gluten:

- Abyssinian Hard (Wheat triticum durum)
- Alcohol (Spirits—Specific Types)
- Amino Acids

[5] https://www.gluten.net/programs/industry-programs/gluten-free-certification-organization/faq-gluten-free-certification-organization-gfco/

[6] http://www.celiac.com/articles/182/1/Unsafe-Gluten-Free-Food-List-Unsafe-Ingredients/Page1.html

- Atta Flour
- Barley Grass (can contain seeds)
- Barley
- Barley Malt
- Beer (most contain barley or wheat)
- Bleached Flour
- Bread Flour
- Brewer's Yeast
- Brown Flour
- Bulgur (Bulgur Wheat/Nuts)
- Bulgur Wheat
- Cereal Binding
- Chilton
- Club Wheat (Triticum aestivum subspecies compactum)
- Common Wheat (Triticum aestivum)
- Cookie Crumbs
- Cookie Dough
- Cookie Dough Pieces
- Couscous
- Crisped Rice
- Dinkle (Spelt)
- Disodium Wheatgermamido Peg-2
- Sulfosuccinate
- Durum wheat (Triticum durum)
- Edible Coatings

- Edible Films
- Edible Starch
- Einkorn (Triticum monococcum)
- Emmer (Triticum dicoccon)
- Enriched Bleached Flour
- Enriched Bleached Wheat Flour
- Enriched Flour
- Farina
- Farina Graham
- Farro
- Filler
- Flour (normally this is wheat)
- Fu (dried wheat gluten)
- Germ
- Graham Flour
- Granary Flour
- Groats (barley, wheat)
- Hard Wheat
- Heeng
- Hing
- Hordeum Vulgare
- Hordeum Vulgare Extract
- Hydroxypropyltrimonium
- Hydrolyzed Wheat Protein
- Kamut (Pasta wheat)

- Kecap Manis (Soy Sauce)
- Ketjap Manis (Soy Sauce)
- Kluski Pasta
- Maida (Indian wheat flour)
- Malt
- Malted Barley Flour
- Malted Milk
- Malt Extract
- Malt Syrup
- Malt Flavoring
- Malt Vinegar
- Macha Wheat (Triticum aestivum)
- Matza
- Matzah
- Matzo
- Matzo Semolina
- Meripro 711
- Mir
- Nishasta
- Oriental Wheat (Triticum turanicum)
- Orzo Pasta
- Pasta
- Pearl Barley
- Persian Wheat (Triticum carthlicum)
- Perungayam

- Poulard Wheat (Triticum turgidum)
- Polish Wheat (Triticum polonicum)
- Rice Malt (if barley or Koji are used)
- Roux
- Rusk
- Rye
- Seitan
- Semolina
- Semolina Triticum
- Shot Wheat (Triticum aestivum)
- Small Spelt
- Spirits (Specific Types)
- Spelt (Triticum spelta)
- Sprouted Wheat or Barley
- Stearyldimoniumhydroxypropyl
- Strong Flour
- Suet in Packets
- Tabbouleh
- Tabouli
- Teriyaki Sauce
- Timopheevi Wheat (Triticum timopheevii)
- Triticale X triticosecale
- Triticum Vulgare (Wheat) Flour Lipids
- Triticum Vulgare (Wheat) Germ Extract
- Triticum Vulgare (Wheat) Germ Oil

- Udon (wheat noodles)
- Unbleached Flour
- Vavilovi Wheat (Triticum aestivum)
- Vital Wheat Gluten
- Wheat, Abyssinian Hard triticum durum
- Wheat
- Wheat Bran Extract
- Wheat, Bulgur
- Wheat Durum Triticum
- Wheat Germ Extract
- Wheat Germ Glycerides
- Wheat Germ Oil
- Wheat Germamidopropyldimonium Hydroxypropyl
- Wheat Grass (can contain seeds)
- Wheat Nuts
- Wheat Protein
- Wheat Triticum aestivum
- Wheat Triticum Monococcum
- Wheat (Triticum Vulgare) Bran Extract
- Whole-Meal Flour
- Wild Einkorn (Triticum boeotictim)
- Wild Emmer (Triticum dicoccoides)

What *Can* I Eat?

Let's go back and look again at what you can eat when you're gluten free. There are plenty of delicious options:

- Corn, grits, polenta and cornmeal (GMO-free is best)
- Buckwheat, buckwheat cereal, kasha and buckwheat flour
- Rice: white, brown, risotto, basmati, jasmine, sticky rice, rice cereal
- Rice flour: white rice, sweet (glutinous) rice and brown rice flour
- Quinoa, quinoa cereal flakes, and quinoa flour
- Millet and millet flour
- Sorghum flour
- Amaranth and amaranth flour
- Certified Gluten-Free oats and oatmeal
- Coconut flour
- Teff flour
- Nut meals and flours—almond, chestnut, pecan, cashew
- Chick pea, garbanzo, soy (soya) and bean flour
- Tapioca (whole) and tapioca starch (manioc)
- Potato starch (used in baking)
- Potato flour (used sparingly as a thickener)
- Sweet potato and yam flour
- Arrowroot starch
- Cornstarch

Add to this list all the fruits and vegetables you love. Then add your favorite proteins. Next remember you may add dairy products if you choose (more on dairy and pain relief soon).

There are many food choices that allow you to be gluten free in a healthy, pain-relieving way. Part Two of this book features practical solutions to all of these questions—meal-by-meal.

My Gluten-Free Story

Countless people out there in the blogosphere and health world are talking about eating gluten free. I've been reading and listening to them for years—have you? Here's a little bit about why I finally chose to go gluten free, and, more importantly, what it did for me. I hope that my story can help you.

As I mentioned earlier, after I was diagnosed with arthritis I frequently heard about the connection between gluten and chronic inflammation. I resisted the change because I grew up loving bread, so being 100% gluten free sounded like a small bit of hell here on earth. But, just in case, I started to eliminate processed breakfast cereals and limit my bread consumption. I still had the occasional pizza or subs, cookies or cakes, but definitely found that the more healthy, clean, unprocessed choices I made, the better I felt. And yet, even at that time, to go completely gluten-free? Nope, I wasn't ready yet.

After a while, though, things started to shift. When I read *The Blood Sugar Solution* by Mark Hyman, M.D., hoping to gain some insight for a newly diabetic family member, the connections really started to click. What? A book about diabetes talked about gluten? Yup—and inflammation—and the connection between the two. I also found an article that seemed credible covering the connection between autoimmunity and gluten. I then read *Why Do I Still Have Thyroid Symptoms? When My Lab Tests Are Normal* by Datis Kharrazian, DHSc, DC, MS, about the connection between thyroid issues, autoimmunity, and gluten. More reading and more credible, scientific connections ensued, and I decided it was time to give gluten-free living a try.

Want to know what flipped the final switch? Well, I just happened to stand on the scale one morning. The previous evening I'd had two small pieces of pizza and a few baked, breaded shrimp. Shocker! The scale showed I had gained four pounds overnight. Nothing else in my food the day before was inflammatory, but four pounds of water/inflammation had packed on from just a moderate serving of wheat-based food. I should mention here that I'm not super worried about my weight—it's healthy and I fit into my clothes, which are regular size for my height. That's another reason why four pounds overnight seemed crazy.

After all of my research I believed there was at least some truth to the connection between gluten and inflammation. I said to myself, "I'll give it 4 to 6 weeks and see how I feel. If there's no change, I can always go back to gluten."

But it didn't take 4 to 6 weeks to see a difference. It took only 4 to 6 *days!* Truthfully, I spent the first several weeks noticing new improvements every couple of days. Again, this is my bio-individual experience. It may be like this for you, but chances are your experience will be different from mine.

Here's what I noticed:

- Flexibility. I noticed this first, and as a massage therapist, this change was extremely helpful. Bonus—it's easier to get on the floor and play with our grandkids.
- Noticeable reduction in morning stiffness, especially in my hands. Again, this is especially helpful when I have early morning massage clients.
- Strength and more muscle soreness. I think keeping my muscles strong will ultimately benefit my joints, so this is important to me. The soreness is an indication that the muscles are more able to strengthen now.

- Major changes in how clothing waistlines fit. I had a small weight change, too, plus every single piece of clothing got looser and all "muffin tops" were gone.
- Feet less swollen at night. I stand for up to 8 hours each day, so this comfort level change is huge.
- Less wildly uncontrollable hunger. I used to say my stomach was really a headless monster, but not anymore!
- Less irritability, especially around hunger. This is huge because I had been attributing irritability to hormone changes, an idea I've begun to question.
- Calmer emotions, even in times of great stress. I'm in the sandwich generation and a small business owner—I need to be calmer every day.
- Less brain fog—not "losing words" or my train of thought at all. This has been super helpful and makes me feel a lot less crazy.
- Less brain fog part two—making goals and planning steps in a way I hadn't done in *years.* Clarity. Focus. Feeling normal again. This is priceless.
- Changes in muscle definition and general tissue quality. Now you can see my muscles, plus they feel looser and less tense to both me and *my* massage therapist.

I can't say for sure that going gluten-free will help you achieve these same improvements, but I wish good changes of any type for you! All the research that I've seen points to gluten as a major pain culprit for MANY of us. That, plus our experiences, makes me hopeful for myself and for you. Doesn't HOPE make all the difference each morning when your feet hit the floor?

"Great-Grandmother Foods"

What's a Great-Grandmother Food?

When it comes to food choices that benefit holistic pain relief efforts, it's important to remember our great-grandparents. As I write this book, I keep a photo of my great-grands on my desk. They inspire me!

Why?

Simple—thinking about great-grandparents makes choosing pain-relieving foods easy. If your great-grandparents wouldn't recognize the ingredients in a food, your body won't either! And choices with lots of food additives and chemicals (unknown to past generations) can increase our pain levels.

I also think about how my great-grandmother shopped. My great-grandparents had a farm, so they grew their own food, and they were farming in a naturally organic way, mostly before the advent of chemical pesticides. They knew the people who raised their meat and produced their dairy. For most of their lives, they didn't even know what a supermarket was. Almost none of their food even *had* labels and ingredient lists—and we can use that as a guide today, too.

If my great-grandmother were shopping at the supermarket today, what would she do with labels? I think she would look for these two main things:

- Are there less than 10 ingredients in this food?
- Can I pronounce every item on the ingredient list, and do I know what the items are?

Those are the two principles I use every time I shop, and that's what I've been teaching my holistic pain relief clients. It's a simple way to take your focus away from processed foods. Remember your great-grandparents!

Food Stories and Memories

Often I'll ask clients if they have any food memories from their childhood. It's amazing the stories we all have to tell, and how they connect to our habits today. For example, I have a food memory that leads directly back to my great-grandparents again. My great-grandmother was a very large figure in my mother's life. They spent summers together at the farm when Mom was very young. That's where Mom learned to make pie—including a super-flaky piecrust. When I was growing up, Mom taught me to make pie—including all the secrets to a flaky and delicious crust.

Even though sweet and gooey pie isn't part of my anti-inflammatory diet today, when I do make a pie for my family, it's out of love. My husband loves blueberry pie, and my granddaughter loves peach pie. As a special treat, we'll make these during the summer with fantastic organic or locally grown fruits. (We've even tried a few gluten-free crust recipes together!)

Because I know it affects my pain levels, I may only have a small sliver or sometimes none at all, but this memory makes me feel connected to the generations before me, and adds another dimension to every pie I've ever made. I especially love teaching my family about my own food memories—it's a small, every day type of legacy to leave behind.

My nutrition mentor, Institute for Integrative Nutrition founder, Joshua Rosenthal, calls this type of experience "primary food." Primary food is what feeds your soul, going way beyond the moments of simply making and eating a meal.

Eating pie with a history of love is so much deeper and more fulfilling than eating a store-bought pie. That feeling of love connections through food is a big part of finding health and pain relief, inside and out.

High Quality Food and Maximizing Nutrition

Whether they knew it or not, our great-grandparents made every calorie as full of fueling nutrition as possible. I don't mean they counted calories, but they had no "empty" calories.

As an example, let's look at a typical lunch meal. I remember my dad packing his lunch every day—I know a lot of us still do. His included a lunchmeat sandwich, milk in a thermos, and maybe a hunk or two of cheese.

I've packed my lunch for work countless times. Twenty years ago I'd make a big container of salad every Sunday, and use it during the week. That salad was iceberg lettuce, carrots, tomatoes, and cucumbers. I'd put some canned tuna on top of it each day and some dressing. Then I'd have an apple as a snack later in the afternoon. Which option offers more fantastic nutrition? And let's note…there are a few things I'd do differently today. (Read: no more iceberg!)

Your body needs nutritious building blocks to function. If you think about food as fuel, you might make different choices. Let's look now at two examples of nutrition you need to help minimize pain. We've probably all heard that muscles need protein to function. In fact, last year I attended a conference called *Women in Pain* (http://www.forgrace.org/women/in/pain_home/). One of the speakers was Forest Tennant, M.D., a renowned pain management specialist. Dr. Tennant strongly advocates a high protein diet for pain relief, whether high quality animal, vegetarian, or vegan. What you gain with high protein is amino acids, which make endorphins (our body's natural painkillers) work.

You also want to be aware that experiencing pain will drive down blood sugar. That's why people in pain find themselves craving sugar or carbs. Adding more protein each day will help balance this blood sugar issue.

Have you ever thought about where to get protein? Or how much protein? Did you know there's protein in many things besides animal meat? For example, by switching my salad's iceberg lettuce for spinach I gain 5 grams of protein for every cup. And when I add 1 tablespoon of hemp seeds on top of that salad I gain 5 more grams.

The International Osteoporosis Foundation recommends we balance the acid-producing nutrients (primarily from meat and cereal grains) with the alkalinizing properties of whole, fresh, vegetables and fruits. This acid/alkaline balance is important for both muscles and bones. It's not that we shouldn't have ANY of the acid-producing foods, but we're out of balance with TOO MANY of them compared to the alkalinizing foods.

In my experience, muscle tension (one of the major sources of chronic pain) is also greatly increased by more acid-producing than alkalinizing foods.

Protein is what's called a macronutrient. But there's another component to nutrition that's super important for holistic pain relief: MICRONUTRIENTS. Micronutrients are the essential phytochemicals, vitamin, and mineral elements in the foods we eat. You've certainly heard about vitamins and minerals, but what about phytochemicals? According to one of my teachers, Joel Fuhrman, M.D.,[7] "Phytochemicals are

[7] Super Immunity: The Essential Nutrition Guide for Boosting Your Body's Defenses to Live Longer, Stronger, and Disease Free, Joel Fuhrman, M.D., HarperOne, 2011.

bioactive, plant-derived chemical compounds important for the growth and survival of the plant…" AND "…the human immune system evolved depending on these phytochemicals for its optimal functioning." You may have heard them discussed by their specific classes: antioxidants, carotenes, bioflavonoids, flavonoids, lignans, and many, many more.

Now, how do you add them to your dietary choices without having to become a scientist? Here's a simple way to remember: GOMBBS. That stands for greens, onions, mushrooms, beans, berries, and seeds. Fuhrman groups these foods together based on many scientific studies. Add these foods into your daily and weekly choices, and you'll automatically be reducing your pain levels and increasing the micronutrients your body has available to heal and improve itself.

Another part of the pain puzzle is bones. Bones need calcium, vitamin D, phosphorus, vitamin A, vitamin C, magnesium, vitamin K, and healthy fats to function. Each of these nutrients offers a different function to our bodies. I think about bone health because when bones aren't strong and healthy, they make small shifts trying to accommodate their weaknesses. Then our soft tissue is out of place—pulled and tugged and stretched to a spot it's not designed to settle into. Then something starts to ache, and the pain cycle begins.

Why not just get all of these micronutrients from supplements? That idea is something called nutritionism, and it has some dangers.

What is nutritionism? Nutritionism is the idea that all you need is the vitamin or mineral to gain the benefit. It began in the twentieth century, when we started to have the scientific equipment and knowledge to separate a food substance into its parts—for example, being able to determine the grams of protein, carbs, or fat in a food. That also led us to finding all of these different vitamins and minerals—and pulling them out of natural or chemical sources to make supplements.

The reason why nutritionism is dangerous, is that we don't know if the benefits from vitamin C, for example, depend on the fiber or other substances in the orange. What about the foods that orange is served with? Might they increase the vitamin C levels or ease of absorption? Is it possible that sharing that orange with someone you love could increase the levels even further? There's no supplement that can replace a day's worth of healthy, nutritious food choices.

Your Takeaway:

- Add in whole foods and minimize processed foods
- Strategize how to cook at home at least 80% of your week
- Listen to what your body needs

Maximizing Smart Nutrition vs. All Those Additives

It turns out that one of my key migraine triggers is MSG (monosodium glutamate)[8], which hides on many ingredient lists with a lot of different names. On top of that, MSG is derived[9] from "natural" ingredients, so it's even in the healthier (but still processed) food choices.

MSG is considered a natural ingredient because of the glutamate. Glutamate in its original form is a component of seaweed—that's how it was discovered—so it can still be added to things that say "Natural" on the front. You may also find some version of glutamate or MSG in organic and organically certified foods.

[8] http://migraine.com/blog/locate-hidden-msg-migraine-triggers/

[9] http://culinaryarts.about.com/od/seasoningflavoring/p/msg.htm

Now, what does all this have to do with the many kinds of food additives[10]? As a holistic health coach, it's not easy for me to admit that I was regularly consuming some gluten-free foods with a lot of additives. I was also making assumptions that food I thought was "whole" wouldn't have harmful ingredients—I had gotten lazy about checking ingredient lists.

Here's an example: Head into the dairy section of your nearest supermarket and look at cottage cheese ingredient lists. Shouldn't they have just a few ingredients—milk, cream, etc.? (Or, as I like to joke—cottage and cheese, right?) The organic, hormone, and antibiotic-free cottage cheese brands have just as many additives as the conventional brands. If you see eight brands on the shelf, you may find only one with the "great-grandmother" ingredient list—less than seven ingredients that only include items your great-grandmother would recognize. Whether you eat dairy or not is a whole separate topic, but if you do, then choose the type with the "great-grandmother" ingredient list.

More importantly, look for ways to incorporate foods WITHOUT ingredient lists and labels. These are the truly whole foods in our lives—food that IS a plant (not food made in manufacturing plants).

Here are some examples of other names for MSG you may see on your food's ingredient list:

- AJI-NO-MOTO®
- Amino Acids
- Anything with the word 'hydrolyzed' including hydrolyzed protein

[10] http://chriskresser.com/?s=harmful+or+harmless

- Anything "...protein," for example "textured protein"
- Autolyzed Yeast
- Calcium Glutamate
- Calcium Caseinate
- Gelatin
- Glutamic Acid
- Glutamate
- Hydrolyzed corn gluten
- Kombu extract
- Magnesium Glutamate
- Monoammonium Glutamate
- Monopotassium Glutamate
- MSG
- Natrium Glutamate
- Natural flavors (may contain up to 20% MSG)
- Seaweed
- Sodium Caseinate
- Soy Protein
- Soy Protein Concentrate
- Soy Protein Isolate
- Textured Protein
- Umami
- Whey Protein
- Whey Protein Concentrate
- Whey Protein Isolate

- Worcestershire sauce
- Vari-Vox chicken pox vaccine
- Vetsin
- Yeast Extract
- Yeast Food
- Yeast Nutrient

If you're sensitive to MSG, you may also be sensitive to free glutamate. Foods that often contain free glutamate, or where free glutamate is created in their processing procedures, include:

- Anything "enzyme modified"
- Anything fermented
- Anything "protein fortified"
- Anything labeled "ultra pasteurized"
- Aspartame
- Barley malt
- Carrageenan
- Citric Acid
- Citrate
- Boullion
- Broth (not from scratch under controlled circumstances)
- Dough conditioners
- Enzymes
- Flavors
- Flavoring
- Guar Gum

- Locust Bean Gum
- Malt Extract
- Malted Barley
- Maltodextrin
- Mushrooms
- Pectin
- Protease
- Sea Salt
- Seasonings
- Soy sauce
- Soy sauce extract
- Soy protein
- Stock (not from scratch under controlled circumstances)
- Wheat protein
- Xanthan Gum

Remember bio-individuality? MSG and other food additives are a perfect example of bio-individual tolerance. Not everyone will have pain-related connections to every food additive, and the way you are impacted by a food additive can shift and change throughout your life. So even though your BFF thinks she can eat all those processed foods, she might someday find that MSG creates an unhealthy situation for her. Or you may need to cut down now on all kinds of MSG, but later on determine that you're really just sensitive to xanthan gum.

Some items on these MSG lists can be super positive for your health and digestion. For example, seaweed in its purest forms can be a fantastic addition to your food choices. Any possible reaction to it, good or bad, is bio-individual.

If this makes your head spin, then *now* is the time to reach out to me or another health or holistic pain relief coach. We are trained to help you filter the facts relevant for your condition, and how to translate the bio-individual information you discover into real life choices.

MSG and Pain

In 2001, a study was published in *The Annals of Pharmacotherapy*[11] that linked consumption of MSG (and aspartame) to fibromyalgia pain. Removing the additives from the diet of people with pre-existing fibromyalgia reduced their pain completely or nearly completely.

Researchers published another study in *Cephalalgia*[12] in 2009 about MSG. They found that men drinking soda with MSG in it experienced a significant increase in headache pain and muscle tenderness in their heads.

At Oregon Health and Sciences University in 2012, researchers published[13] results of a study that connected a 30%+ decrease in symptoms with removal of MSG from the diet of study participants.

These all seem to me like pretty good reasons for change! It's not always easy to figure out which foods include MSG, and when you eat out, you can't always control everything in your food. But when you live with chronic pain, wouldn't you try

[11] http://aop.sagepub.com/content/35/6/702.short

[12] http://onlinelibrary.wiley.com/doi/10.1111/j.1468-2982.2009.01881.x/abstract

[13] http://europepmc.org/abstract/MED/22766026

just about anything to get relief? I know that's exactly how I felt when the migraine activity was at its worst.

MSG is Addictive!

If these reasons aren't enough for you, let me give you one more. Like gluten, MSG has addictive properties. Eating MSG can damage[14] the part of your brain where the leptin receptors lie. Leptin receptors tell your brain when you've had enough food. They tell you to stop eating. And if MSG damages those receptors, it's contributing to our need for ever-growing portion sizes.

If we're trying to cut back on MSG for pain-related reasons, eating even the smallest bit can encourage us to eat more—and feel more pain! This is really tough to hear, I know, but when you try reducing your consumption for a time, I think you'll find it's worth continuing.

[14] http://ajpendo.physiology.org/content/273/1/E202
http://www.sciencedirect.com/science/article/pii/S0083672900590104

Dairy Products and Holistic Pain Relief

When I was a kid I hated the taste of milk. There aren't many things I'd use the word "hate" for, but I did (and still do) hate milk. Unfortunately for me, my dad loved milk. He drank almost two gallons of skim milk every week throughout his life. As a kid, I was required to drink a glass of milk with every meal, but some days I simply couldn't stomach another glass. I'd eat my whole meal, never touching the milk. Maybe I thought it would magically disappear, or that somehow I'd be off the hook, but that magic never happened for me.

One night when I was about eight years old, I was avoiding my milk, hoping it would magically disappear. At the end of the meal, Dad said I had to stay at the table until my milk glass was empty. I sat and stared at that full glass, and it stared back at me. It got warmer and warmer with each passing minute. Then Dad added ice cubes, because I used the warmth as an excuse to stop drinking. Of course now it was an even worse situation. Skim milk is thin and skim milk with melting ice is utterly horrible. I finally had to drink the wretched stuff, and as soon as I had a choice about beverages, I stopped drinking glasses of milk.

Since becoming a health coach, I've started to wonder if my childhood self had an innate sense of what was really healthy for me. As an adult I've learned that dairy is painfully disruptive to my digestion, and inflammatory to my body. No matter your feelings about dairy foods, I'd like to help you learn about their connection to pain.

What's Inflammatory About Dairy?

The conventional methods of processing and pasteurization (heating at high temperatures) de-natures[15] the protein, fat, and calcium considered the beneficial elements of dairy products. Thus, they're also generally inflammatory to our bodies.

Conventionally produced cow's milk contains xenoestrogens, synthetic growth hormones, and antibiotics. These are all substances that can cause inflammation in our bodies.

The marketing engine for dairy products will never tell us we don't actually need dairy products to survive. You can get all of the elements mentioned above—calcium, protein and fat—from alternate dietary sources. For example, dark green leafy vegetables are one of the richest (and most untapped) sources of calcium available.

Another inflammatory issue with dairy items like cheese and ice cream, is the way milk is super-concentrated to make them. Imagine not just one "layer" of milk, but many more "layers" or concentrations. So, if you have an inflammatory connection to milk, it may actually be even more difficult for your body to manage its highly concentrated forms.

Many food items we think of as dairy products are also loaded with sugar—things like yogurt, frozen yogurt, and ice cream. That's another strong inflammatory connection since sugar and pain are closely linked.

[15] http://www.realmilk.com/health/pasteurization-does-harm-real-milk/

Cheeses that are the most inflammatory are those with mold, such as blue cheese, and soft varieties such as Brie. Also if you're migraine-sensitive like I am, the harder cheeses, such as Parmesan and cheddar, can also be inflammatory due to their aging process. Molds used in blue and other cheeses are essentially a toxin to our bodies. They set off your natural defense system, creating inflammation to "protect" you from that toxin. Remember, a little inflammation for a short period of time IS protective. Inflammation leading to chronic pain is caused by long-term, high-volume ingestion of substances our body doesn't recognize and doesn't understand—so it will constantly "protect" us by creating increased inflammation.

Practical Strategy

Like many of the inflammatory foods listed earlier, dairy can be hidden on ingredient lists with alternate names. This will be especially useful if you're not getting the pain relief you hoped for by removing dairy from your diet. Some dairy-related ingredients include:

- Casein
- Hydrolyzed whey protein
- Lactablumin
- Lactalbumin phosphate
- Lactic acid
- Lactoglobulin
- Lactose
- Simplesse
- Whey
- Whey protein isolate
- Whey powder

Steps to Reducing Dairy Consumption

Let's consider some steps you can take to start incorporating these ideas. As I always say, pick one step at a time. Once you've integrated that change into your life, pick another step.

As you're beginning to reduce dairy, there's some possibility that you may find organic, grass-fed, naturally raised dairy to be less inflammatory and more tolerable. You may want to test these products after eliminating all conventionally produced dairy for at least a week or two.

You can also opt for many non-dairy beverages available to you at the supermarket. Almond, oat, rice, and hemp "milks" are all examples of non-dairy beverages. I caution you, however, to read the labels on these or any milk substitutes. They often contain carrageenan, which contains free glutamate (MSG) that can be inflammatory.

Try some easy substitutions for dairy in your cooking. For example:

- A cup of broth can replace milk in a savory recipe.
- Pureed sweet potato or coconut milk make recipes creamier.
- With a sweet recipe, you can use a non-dairy milk in equal quantities to the suggested cow's milk.
- When you're baking, add a tablespoon of healthy, non-inflammatory oil to maintain the richness and consistency of a recipe.

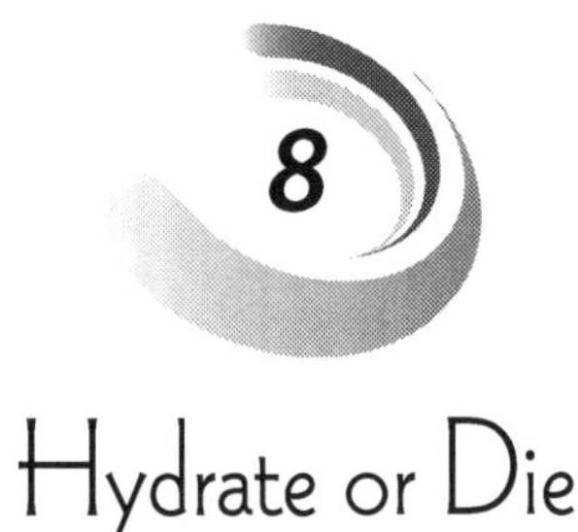

Hydrate or Die

Being properly hydrated is critical to many aspects of wellness, and holistic pain relief in particular. The big question is, what does "properly hydrated" mean to you?

Back in 2008, I had the opportunity to participate as a support team member during the bicycling race called Race Across America or RAAM. I was the massage therapist for a team of four cyclists and eight crew members. The race began in mid-June on the West Coast—beautiful Oceanside, California. We traveled to the finish in Annapolis, Maryland in just over seven days. The cyclists rode as a relay without stopping for overnight resting periods. In fact, none of us had normal sleep for the entire race. We just grabbed our zzzz's as we could, rotating crew and cyclist duties to continue moving forward. It was one of the most physically challenging events I've ever participated in—as much for our crew as our cyclists.

You're wondering what this has to do with hydration, right? Well, that's when the phrase, "hydrate or die" became a part of my regular vocabulary. We went through California's famous Death Valley, and hydration was equally essential on every other day of our eight-day journey. Riders and crew were pushing themselves to the limits of physical and mental endurance. We had almost no time to eat a proper meal, but fuel was critical, so we grabbed healthy food as we could. No matter the food choices, we *always* made sure water was available for everyone.

If you're living with chronic pain, the importance of hydration cannot be overstated. Not one system in your body—muscles, bones, blood, lungs, heart, digestion, etc.—can work correctly if it doesn't have enough fluid. The water we drink supplies that fluid.

Think about your pain, whether muscle tension, headache, or something else, as a communication from your body. Often pain is a cry for hydration—more water!

How Much Water is Enough?

You probably grew up with the message I did, "Eight 8 oz. glasses of water a day is best," but there has been some disagreement about whether this advice is logical for all of us, as hydration, like so many other aspects of our health needs, is bio-individual.

I recommend letting two things be your guide: thirst, and urine color. These two indicators are a simple way to tell what your body is communicating. When you're thirsty, you may already be dehydrated, so drink water; and know that you may need more than one glass. You may need well more than eight ounces, and that's where having a refillable water bottle can be so helpful. They are larger and often designed to keep water cool if you prefer it that way. When you're dehydrated, your urine will be dark yellow or almost orange/brown. That's another cue to drink more water. The more hydrated you generally are, the easier it will be to change that urine color back to clear. If you've been dehydrated for a long time, it may take more time and water to change the color[16]. Let your body teach you the best amount for you, adjusting for conditions like heat and activity level.

[16] http://chriskresser.com/hydration-101-how-much-water-do-you-really-need

Will Other Liquids Hydrate Like Water?

The short answer is no. Somewhere in the last few decades, we've decided that water doesn't have enough taste. It's not as interesting to our palate as some other options, especially the multi-flavored soda and energy drink concoctions we see on shelves today. So we choose coffee, tea, soda, energy drinks, juice—there are a multitude of options!

Many of these beverages contain caffeine, which actually dehydrates your body. Caffeine flushes water *out* of the system, which is exactly the effect we need to avoid. I'm not saying you have to completely eliminate caffeine (although that's something to consider), but if you're living with chronic pain, it may not be helping your body feel better. The choice is always yours.

Additives In Your Water

Did you know that some bottled waters[17] have added ingredients? Some include magnesium sulfate, potassium chloride, and salt. These ingredients serve no useful purpose for our bodies. They don't increase hydration; in fact, they will most likely make you *more* thirsty so you drink more of that expensive water.

Some bottled water is actually just tap water. This is such a lesson in why reading ingredient lists is important. We cannot ever assume that anything is "just" the name on the label, especially when we live with chronic pain. There are many filtering options available that can be attached to your home's tap water. You can investigate the quality of your municipal water—I receive a report in the mail from my municipality about water quality.

[17] http://wellnessandequality.com/2014/02/19/dasani-bottled-water-has-4-ingredients-tap-water-known-teratogen-lethal-drug-and-salt/

Hydration Strategy

Here's a simple way to be sure you get enough hydration. First, buy 4–5 refillable water bottles and mark each of them with a different interval during the day. I recommend using glass or stainless steel bottles to reduce your exposure to pain-creating toxins. So one says 8 AM–11 AM, and the next says 11 AM–1 PM, 1 PM–5 PM, 5 PM–10 PM. Use the intervals that work with your sleeping and waking cycle during the day. Start the first one immediately upon waking.

When the first bottle is empty then you move on to the next and so on. And notice that the intervals between them are shorter in the morning. Drinking more water in the morning helps detoxify us, and also means we're less likely to have to get up in the middle of the night for the bathroom.

If you find that carrying multiple bottles of water is impractical in your day, set some timers on your phone as reminders. Name the timer something like, "Have you finished 24 oz. of water since 8 AM?"

9 Supplements

You may ask where I stand on supplements as part of a holistic pain relief plan. I've certainly taken my share of supplements over the years. However, supplements are not the *foundation* of a holistic pain relief plan, they are simply an important part of the overall structure.

Supplements can help ensure that you're not missing vital nutrients, but they're not designed to *be* the vital nutrients in your diet. Incorporating nutritious, non-processed foods in your diet is the first foundation of holistic pain relief. Removing the pain-creating foods we've discussed here is the next foundation. Beyond that, you may find that a few supplements are helpful for your pain relief. Your choices will vary, because like with food, your needs are bio-individual.

You'll want to find a local store with a broad selection of supplement choices; then start getting to know the staff. Ask detailed questions about their selection. Soon you'll learn who's knowledgeable and able to steer you in the right direction.

I respectfully encourage you to find a multi-vitamin that makes you feel better. Multi-vitamins come in various forms: liquid, tablet, powder. They can also have ingredients beyond vitamins and minerals, like probiotics or super foods. You'll want to consider supplements like magnesium citrate, CoQ10, and a quality greens powder. Of course, any choice you make should be reviewed with your health care provider and healing team.

Part Two

Integrating Changes into Your Life

Putting Suggestions Into Action

What Are Your Motivators to Change?

Just last week I was speaking with a client who has worked with me for about two months. When she first came in, it was hard for her to grip the handlebars on her bicycle. She loves to ride, though, as it helps her mood and her arthritis. After just six weeks of gluten-free and pain-relieving choices, she told me that the reduction in pain was enough to keep her persistent and motivated. Gripping the handlebars on her bike is no problem for her now!

The world of medical care we are used to fosters a mentality of "quick fix", especially if a pill can be given to "solve" a problem. Many people living with chronic pain have used this approach and system for many years, but often find it unsatisfying and frustrating—mostly because the pills don't always work.

People with chronic pain also look outside the medical system to alternative healers, and many healers in both systems encourage an approach where they want to be responsible for someone's well being. Frankly, it's job security—even if it might not help the client or patient escape the "fix me" mentality.

There are also many people living with chronic pain—patients and clients—who want to participate in the healing process. They've found being present and working together with the healer brings better results in the long-term. But it takes a mindset shift from the patient to begin this process.

What are the goals and incentives that would keep you motivated? I suggest starting a journal and putting your goals on the first page. My journal is a hardbound, blank book with lines on the pages. I record what I eat and the symptoms I experience each day. I also track things that affect my pain, like hormones, weather, emotions, and work-related activity. I note the times I have symptoms. Plus, I find it motivating to also note the days I don't have any symptoms at all. It seems intensely detailed, I know, but keeping track of my routines and habits helps me find the valuable connections between what I eat and how I feel.

You can also try one of the many apps and websites available to track what you're eating each day, but the apps don't have every feature to measure everything, which is why I went back to the old-fashioned written journal.

Start With Improving One Meal Each Day

Making holistic pain relieving changes is a big decision. It's an individual choice and you essentially have two ways to approach it. You can eliminate gluten, processed, and pain-creating foods in one meal every day (breakfast, for example), and after you get comfortable with those early change choices, increase the number of meals you eat for pain relief each day.

Another option is, you can choose a short period of time (like 3–4 weeks) and completely eliminate gluten, processed, and pain-creating foods to see if the changes make a difference in your pain levels.

I think that after your short test period, you'll decide to make the changes permanent because you're feeling so good.

So, let's say you're going to start with one meal each day. That's what I did, initially, and my choice was breakfast. In fact, the only reason I have any kind breakfast cereal in the house today is for other people or to use in homemade granola bars. And, of course, it's all gluten free now.

Lastly, I'll take you through a variety of meal options here, so you can get a feel for how it might work for you! But first we have to spend a little time thinking about what happens when you're food shopping.

Grocery Store

Reading Labels

I think label reading has gotten massively overcomplicated in the last several years. It feels like we need a degree in nutrition to understand all the data we have at our fingertips. Believe me, I'm a big fan of having that data available, but it can feel overwhelming.

Because I understand this, let's break labels down into a couple of shorter components. Use the suggestions on this list when you read a label and you'll be in good pain-relieving shape.

- Does this food have no label because it's fruit or vegetable?
- Are there less than 10 ingredients listed?
- Can I easily pronounce everything on the ingredient list?
- Does the allergens list include wheat or dairy?
- Are there any possible MSG ingredients here?

If the food label answers all these questions for you, then you'll know whether or not to put it in your cart.

Using Apps and Smartphones

I love my smartphone and having it makes a difference in my chronic pain relief. So, it's only natural I should have some strategies to recommend to clients, family and friends.

Here are my top tips for you:

Use the browser:

Yes, I am the person in the supermarket aisle who has their phone out and is standing there reading it. No, I'm not on Facebook or texting friends. I'm looking on the Internet for more information about a food or an ingredient. And I'm so grateful to have this option!

What I've done is bookmark a few sites that list "hidden ingredient" names for both gluten and MSG. Here are my favorites:

> http://www.celiac.com/articles/182/1/Unsafe-Gluten-Free-Food-List-Unsafe-Ingredients/Page1.htm
>
> http://migraine.com/blog/locate-hidden-msg-migraine-triggers/
>
> http://www.purezing.com/living/toxins/living_toxins_containsmsg.html

I use the lists online to compare with ingredients I may not be sure about on a food label. I can't tell you how many times this has kept me from buying something that would have later caused me more discomfort.

If, after reviewing my lists, I still want more information I will search "what is polysorbate 80?"—or whatever the mystery ingredient is that day. Sometimes that detail is very helpful.

ShopWell app:

How do you know if foods have gluten, dairy, or other pain-creating ingredients in them? This is the app for you! You can set up your profile preferences to include gluten-free (along with many other dietary considerations), and then just scan the bar codes of food items in the store. I've also found this helpful in assessing items in my clients' kitchens when we're working together.

Marketing vs. Nutrition

Maybe it's because I spent fifteen+ years working in marketing, but my family says I'm "the buzzkill" about nutrition claims on packages. What happens is this: someone says they think a new product is delicious and nutritious, but when I look at the label I'll find several things that aren't as healthy as they thought.

It must be the cynic inside me, but I just don't believe the marketing spin of processed food products today. I am here to *own* my buzzkill vibe because I believe this attitude will keep me healthy and pain free for a long, long time.

Items that need a little buzzkill in my book:

- The fast food chains, especially [insert your favorite here]
- All processed food items sold in a bag or a box
- Comfort foods that don't make our pain (or our guilt complexes) more bearable

Food companies survive on your gullibility and your desire "not to know" what's really going into your body.

Is that the way you'll live your *best* life?

I support your right to choose whatever food you prefer. I only encourage you to be mindful: Spend 2 minutes reading that label or Googling the ingredients of your favorite chicken strips. And *then* choose what you consume.

If ignoring the truth gives you a buzz, I'll pass on that buzz.

My buzz is feeling so much energy that I can skip the afternoon nap.

My buzz is craving exercise and laughter instead of cookies.

My buzz is making choices today that will enable me to feel this pain free in thirty more years.

I choose not to let mindlessness hinder the fullness of life I deserve to experience.

What buzz do you choose—mindful or mindless?

Breakfast

Now that we've covered some of the basics of shopping and food choices, let's think about holistic pain relief and breakfast.

Nine Reasons Why Smoothies are a Delicious, Nutritious Breakfast

Smoothies are one of my favorite natural remedies for pain relief. I've been having them at breakfast for 10+ years. Here are nine reasons why I recommend you start having smoothies for or with your morning meal:

1. **You can make them in 5 minutes:** You just need a blender and ingredients. The preparation is super quick and easy.
2. **They're anti-inflammatory and help relieve pain:** Smoothies are naturally grain-free and gluten-free, which makes them a wonderful anti-inflammatory choice.
3. **You can pack every bite with TONS of nutrition:** So many super foods are the perfect fit with a smoothie. For example, add some organic blueberries and a teaspoon of cinnamon, turmeric, or ginger. Fantastic for you and so easy!
4. **You'll never miss the gluten or dairy:** Switching the milk or yogurt for non-dairy milk doesn't change the taste at all. You'll never miss it.

5. **They help your digestion:** Having a liquid breakfast is easy on your body. It allows overnight digestion to continue during the morning.
6. **You can save a cup of smoothie for after dinner:** If you love a little something sweet at night, just make some extra smoothie and refrigerate it in a glass jar. Healthy and yummy dessert!
7. **Even kids like them and you can hide a vegetable serving in there for them:** My teenage granddaughter just told me the other day that she has a smoothie in the morning now. Her mom puts kale in it, and my granddaughter says, "You can't even tell!"
8. **If you *must* eat in the car, you can drink your smoothie:** I'd rather eat my smoothie while sitting still at my dining room table, but if your morning routine is crazy, make it a little thinner and take it in the car. You'll still gain plenty of benefits.
9. **It's hydration the easy way:** Many mornings I use mostly or completely water (instead of a non-dairy milk substitute) in my smoothie. Filtered water is always best. Every bit of extra hydration we can get is a boost for pain relief.

BONUS: There are so many flavor options that you'll never get tired of breakfast smoothies.

Practical Strategy

As you're experimenting with smoothie ingredients, you may discover that your smoothie has turned brown and isn't very appetizing. This is because red (like strawberries) and green (like kale) mix together to make brown. The taste may still be terrific, but you'll never talk a teenager (or the teen inside you) into eating that smoothie.

My easy solution is to add raw cacao powder. Cacao is the raw ingredient for chocolate, so you're really just turning that accidentally brown smoothie into a chocolate flavor surprise. Cacao has many health benefits but can also be a tad bitter, so be careful with the amount. I like to add about two teaspoons.

Here's my favorite smoothie recipe:

Blueberry Energy Surprise

Ingredients:

1 cup almond milk

½ cup organic greens (spinach or kale are favorites, but sometimes I use romaine lettuce if that's what I have)

2 tablespoons each, freshly ground chia seeds and flax seeds

1 ½ tablespoons vegan protein

1 banana or 3 pitted, dried dates

⅓ to ½ avocado

½ cup frozen, organic blueberries

Dash of cinnamon

½ teaspoon pure vanilla extract

1. Put everything in the blender in the order above and blend until smooth: About 30–60 seconds.
2. Enjoy a rich, thick, tasty smoothie every morning!

No gluten, dairy or other pain-creating foods. Nothing but valuable nutrients that give you fantastic fuel for your day.

Now, here's the rationale behind each ingredient:

Almond milk is easier on your body than dairy milk or yogurt—again, it's a pain-relieving choice. You can substitute whatever non-dairy milk you prefer.

The minerals in the greens are important energy building blocks for your body. These building blocks also help your body repair cellular damage.

Chia and flax are both rich in fiber and omega-3 fatty acids, which are anti-inflammatory. I grind the seeds in a small coffee grinder just before adding them to my smoothie. (I don't grind coffee in that grinder!)

Vegan protein is better for your thyroid than soy, and again, it's non-dairy. Most vegan protein is made from ingredients like brown rice and peas.

Bananas or dates give you a bit of natural sweetness and some great nutrients. If you're watching your sugar intake, you may want to reduce the amount.

Avocado is a high-quality healthy fat option, giving you more omega-3s, and it thickens the smoothie like nobody's business.

Blueberries are antioxidants that keep your body from oxidizing (rusting). And I believe a less rusty body is going to hurt less, don't you?

Cinnamon is anti-inflammatory and good for blood pressure among other things, and the vanilla is purely a taste booster—it balances the bitter of the greens.

Lunch

Lunch can be a challenge because many of us are at work during the day. Lunch "hour" isn't always an actual 60-minute time period, and sometimes we have work-related obligations like lunch with colleagues, customers, or the boss.

As you begin this holistic pain relief way of life, you may find it easier to pack your lunch. Salad is my go-to choice for lunch. When you go with salad, you can vary the selection of vegetables to keep things tasty and interesting. Often I'll make enough salad to last for a few days as a time saver. Each day I'll add leftover protein from dinner the night before. I also make my own simple oil and vinegar dressings to lessen pain-causing processed food ingredients. These are time saving tips that make a healthy routine simple and fast Monday to Friday.

A few years ago, Cris wanted to lose some weight and make healthier choices. But he was working in sales and on the road up to eight hours each day. Although he loves to stop in locally owned restaurants, we also targeted his most likely fast food stops. For each of those chains, we reviewed the menu's nutritional information available online. It was pretty eye opening! For example, at one fast food chain we found that the items with the most trans fats were actually the "healthy" choices. No matter how healthy they were, trans fats don't benefit a pain-relieving lifestyle. We were able to make some good and better choices for Cris to achieve his goals. It's a wonderful thing to have this information available—and well worth making some time to take advantage of the opportunity!

Another practical option: Gather take out menus from your favorite lunch spots. Spread them out and assess which menu choices are the most likely to support your pain-relieving efforts. You may also want to use this chance to check out some different restaurant choices in your area—maybe you'll find some pain-relieving menu options you hadn't anticipated.

Practical Strategy

If you're like me, you like to end lunch with a bit of sweetness, but heading to the office candy machine for dessert is counter-productive to your pain-relieving goals, isn't it? I recommend packing some healthy dessert and snack options in your lunch bag. My favorite options are in Chapter 14: Snacks, and Chapter 16: Desserts.

Marinated Kale Salad

Kale is one of the sweetest greens and a good place to start if you're trying to add more greens to your diet. This salad is easy to make, delicious, and keeps well in the refrigerator. A kale salad like this is much richer in minerals than a typical salad, and more satisfying, too. It can also be modified with a variety of ingredients based on what you have on hand.

Salad:

1 bunch kale (dinosaur or curly types both work), center stems removed, ripped or chopped into bite size pieces

Onions: red onion, very thinly sliced—or chives, shallots or green onions

Vegetables: zucchini, yellow squash or whatever fresh choice is on hand

Fruit: especially good with gala or other sweet apples, in small chunks

Beans: cooked lentils or garbanzo beans go especially well with kale

Avocados, to taste and in small chunks

Marinade:

¾ cup olive or flax oil

Up to ½ cup lemon juice (add just before serving the salad)

1 teaspoon Celtic sea salt

⅛ teaspoon cayenne pepper (add after massaging the salad)

1 clove garlic, crushed (optional)

1. Pour olive or flax oil right onto torn kale leaves, and sprinkle with sea salt. Use your hands to massage and squeeze the kale. This works the salt and oil in and helps make the kale tender. Continue kneading the salad until the kale begins to soften.
2. Before serving, add the diced vegetables, fruit, avocado, beans, cayenne, and garlic.
3. Do not add the lemon juice until just before you eat, as it will change the kale from "fresh green" to an "army green." Mix well, serve, and enjoy!

This salad gets better as it sits. If you plan to keep leftovers, you may want to separate them before adding lemon juice and serving. Leftover salad will generally last up to 3 days in the refrigerator.

Spring Vegetable and Chicken Soup

Soup is a favorite of mine, and this is a great way to have lunch all ready for the week. I often make a pot of soup during the weekend and pack it up for lunches. You can vary vegetable choices based on what's in your kitchen or what's freshest at the market.

1 tablespoon olive oil

2 onions, peeled and chopped

2 cloves garlic, minced

1 teaspoon cumin

2 cups (or 1 can) cooked white beans

1 teaspoon dried basil

3–4 cups mixed spring vegetables (yellow and green squash, green beans, carrots) cut into ¾ inch chunks

2–3 cups chopped kale, leaves only (stems removed)

4 chicken thighs, baked ahead and boned, chopped into ¾ inch chunks

6 cups bean cooking liquid, vegetable stock, or water

Sea salt to taste

1. Heat oil in a large soup pot over medium heat. Add onions and sauté over medium heat for about 10 minutes or until softened and translucent. Add garlic and cumin and sauté for an additional 2 minutes.
2. Add cooked chicken and beans, basil, vegetables, kale, and cooking liquid. Bring to a boil, reduce heat, add salt, and cook for 20 minutes until carrots and squash are tender.
3. Taste and adjust seasoning.

Snacks

As of 2007, Americans spent about $24 billion a year on snacks alone, according to *The Seattle Times.* Figuring there are approximately 300 million Americans, that's about $80 per person, per year.

I'd be way off base if I didn't give you a strategy for choosing pain relieving snacks, because they're obviously a part of our lives. In fact, they're often part of the stuff we call comfort foods. But...

Comfort foods don't make you comfortable!
Did you ever come up with those funny sayings that justify an unhealthy choice? I once knew a guy who'd say, "If it's broken in half, all the calories fall out!" Well, here's one saying we often fall victim to: "Since snacks are in between meals, it doesn't matter if they're healthy, right?"

You're probably thinking you can let your guard down because you'll get right back on the anti-inflammatory track at your next meal. But do you really get back on track? Did that "harmless" snack choice actually harm your pain relief efforts?

The challenge with snacking is two things: what you choose and how much you eat. With today's processed food choices, it's not out of the question to consume an entire day's calories in just one afternoon snack. Wait, what? Why am I talking about calories? No, I don't intend to get caught up in calorie counting. I'm just saying that portion size and quality of nutrition are pretty much non-existent in typical snack choices today.

Instead of counting calories, you may want to count chemicals. How many chemical ingredients are in that snack food? Remember, the chemicals in the food are often what create additional inflammation and pain in your body. So again, the message is: comfort foods don't make you comfortable!

If you're looking for a snack that'll give you more sustained energy, find options with lower carbohydrates and sugar. For example, pair something with natural sugars, like an apple with a protein or fat like a nut butter. This will give you a pain relieving, positive energy balance of carbs, fats, and protein.

You may also find that whether you eat snacks regularly or not is bio-individual. You may find your blood sugar dropping, your energy waning, and your tummy growling more often than others. Heed the call of your body's true signs in regard to snacking. If it's 3:00 in the afternoon and you need something to do for a break, that's appetite, but when your stomach feels empty and you know that dinner is hours away, that's hunger. Use true hunger as your cue for snacking.

Most of the foods we turn to for comfort have ingredients that promote inflammation, and therefore, pain. These include trans fats (partially hydrogenated oils), white sugar and similar sweeteners, wheat flour and gluten, and dairy (for some of us). When you're feeling well and energetic, make time to cultivate an appreciation for a new, healthier style of snack foods. Switch to fresh fruit instead of store-bought cookies. Choose naturally salty foods, like a few olives instead of handfuls of chips. Taking small steps to readjust your taste buds will help you make less pain-creating choices when you're seeking comfort foods.

Practical Strategy

Most snacks are consumed without us giving them any thought. You grab that bag of chips and before you realize it, the entire bag is gone. I *want* you to snack if you need it, but the solution to mindless snacking is planning and paying attention.

First, you have to plan healthy snacks and keep them easily accessible. Then, challenge yourself: stop and eat that snack with attention and mindfulness. Don't do this while driving in the car—it doesn't count! Stop and do nothing else when you try this challenge. Can you pay attention to every bite of that apple? Stop and think about the way the crunch of the first bite feels. Chew it slowly and completely. Really focus on the flavor—tart, sweet, or in between? Take a full breath in between each bite. Think about the way apples grow on trees. How they are picked each fall. Relive any happy memories associated with apples. Even stop for a moment and appreciate your surroundings before biting the apple again. Is it juicy? Shake a bit of cinnamon on the flesh of the apple. How does that enhance the taste?

All of a sudden, you've mindfully and slowly enjoyed your apple. Do you feel more satisfied? Have you had a break—mentally, emotionally and physically? Does it feel like you've been *fed?*

These are great principles for any meal, but they're extra meaningful with snacks. Take a moment to savor your snacks—your body will thank you!

Pain Relieving Snack Ideas

- Whole and/or cut up fruit
- Hummus with carrot sticks, celery, and sliced cucumbers
- Edamame with sea salt and optional lemon

- Non-dairy yogurt with fruit
- Banana dipped into cashew butter, almond butter, or sunflower seed butter
- Kale chips
- Popcorn (homemade, non-microwave, non-GMO)
- Olives
- Nuts, especially almonds and walnuts

Anti-Inflammatory Energy Truffles

Adding anti-inflammatory spices to your foods is an easy boost to your pain relief plan. My favorites are cayenne pepper, cinnamon, ginger, and turmeric. Here's a delicious, fantastically fueling snack that incorporates all four!

Ingredients:

1 cup raw almonds

6 pitted Medjool dates

¼ cup unsweetened flaked or shredded coconut

¼ cup almond butter

⅛ cup coconut oil

2 tablespoons raw honey (optional)

2 tablespoons carob or raw cacao powder

½ teaspoon cinnamon

¼ teaspoon ginger

¼ teaspoon turmeric

Pinch of cayenne pepper (to taste)

1. Put almonds in food processor and process to a medium fine powder. Remove from food processor to a separate bowl.
2. Process pitted dates and flaked coconut together to form a paste.

3. Return almonds to the food processor and add all of the other ingredients. Process until mixture is a smooth paste.
4. Add a bit of non-dairy milk or coconut oil if mix is too dry.
5. Remove from food processor and form into small balls. Roll in carob powder or coconut if desired.

Stored in refrigerator, truffles will keep for one week.

Each truffle is 80–90 calories, and every calorie is packed with nutrients and pain-relieving value. They make a delicious snack; plus, you won't find yourself eating more than a couple at a time because they're also rich and satisfying.

Dinner

When you're planning dinners with holistic pain relief in mind, one thing you want to consider is the quality of the foods you eat. Thinking back to the idea of incorporating "great-grandmother foods," I encourage you to add as many organic foods as possible. It's simple—look for the produce labels that start with the number nine and have a five-digit code. Of course, you want to do this in every meal, but dinner is the perfect place to begin and mention for reference.

Why would choosing organic and non-GMO foods help relieve your pain? Because your body is unfamiliar with genetically modified foods, and when it encounters something unfamiliar, it will increase mucus production. This type of mucus isn't the kind of mucus you see. It's mucus hidden deep within your body (think "boogers" in your body—yuck!), and it's designed to protect your body from the unfamiliar elements of these foods. The more mucus your body makes, the more inflamed you become. The more inflamed you are, the more pain you're likely to experience. This is simply another example of your body's natural, healthy protective responses taken to an extreme that feels uncomfortable and painful.

Why Choose Organic Foods?

The Organic Facts

Why buy organic produce? Because the health benefits, especially for our children, are undeniable. It's as simple as that. Did you know that as of 2008, the U.S. government no longer tests pesticide levels on fruits and vegetables?[18] Commercially-produced crops are not tested or required to adhere to any pesticide standards.

Conventionally or chemically produced crops are damaging your health every day. These crops include pesticides that are endocrine-disruptors and may be affecting your reproductive system, neuroendocrinology, thyroid, and cardiovascular systems. These damages can be passed through your genetics to future generations!

The Endocrine Society has validated the "low-dose response factor." This states that a long-term low dose exposure to chemicals is more harmful than exposure to short term larger doses. So, when conventional food producers say that a small amount of pesticides is not harmful, they aren't telling us the whole story. Organic growing methods include absolutely no harmful chemicals in any dose.

You've probably heard of the weed-killing chemical called Roundup. You may even use it in your own yard or garden. It's used extensively in growing conventional produce. Roundup includes a type of chemical called surfactants that allow it to get INSIDE the food we eat. These chemicals are fat-soluble and every cell in our body is a fatty membrane. They are designed to penetrate every cell of our bodies, and you cannot wash them off. Scary, isn't it?

How to Find Organic Produce Near You

You can find organic produce at:

- Farmer's markets (ask each stand holder if they have organic options)

[18] Organic Manifesto: How Organic Farming Can Heal Our Planet, Feed the World, and Keep Us Safe. Maria Rodale, Rodale Press, 2010

Global News Services, "USDA Halts Pesticide Testing," Morning Call, October 1, 2008, A8.

- Community supported agriculture (CSA) farms
- Local grocery stores or co-ops

You'll also find sources near you by searching at www.localharvest.org or asking your holistic health or pain relief coach!

Practical Strategy

Many people are concerned with the extra costs involved in buying organic produce. But, honestly, it's not as challenging as you think.

If you're worrying about cost, simply start by buying these four products organically—apples, celery, cherry tomatoes, and cucumbers. Why? Because they're the most heavily contaminated with pesticides.

And don't worry so much about finding organic options for these five products—cabbage, avocado, cantaloupe, sweet corn, and asparagus. They're the least heavily contaminated produce items; although you'll want to be aware most sweet corn is GMO.

The Environmental Working Group updates these organic options each year. You can get the latest list here: http://www.ewg.org.

Practical Strategy #2

Dinner is so packed with pitfalls that I'm going to cover one more. And it's a biggie! The pitfall is time—that feeling when you get home and no dinner is made. You're exhausted from your day and can't help but wish for your own personal chef!

One of my favorite food books is by Mark Bittman. It's called *Cooking Solves Everything*. Part of what Bittman does is make some simple connections between how to stock your pantry, and quick dinners you can make anytime. Here's how I suggest you apply these principles:

Keep your pantry stocked with cooking essentials—flavors you like, whole foods that are good in a pinch, basic veggies, and healthy gluten-free grains. Don't let it get bare because that's the first part of the pitfall.

Create 3–4 meals that you and your family love. These should be versatile—meaning you can change the protein, veggies and flavors. But, basically they're the same meal. At our house the menu might be roast, rice, gravy, and veggies. The roast can be chicken, beef, or pork. The veggies are whatever we got at the farmer's market that week. We make sure that vegetables are the largest portion on our plates, then protein, followed by the gluten-free, whole grains.

Your family might prefer to choose a different "favorite meal"—like omelets, stir-fry, or fried rice. One of my clients applies these principles to make a quiche every week for her family. Whatever you find easy to cook and delicious to eat is what works.

One thing I love about the roast combo that we use is how versatile it is for either lunch the next day or leftovers the next night.

This is another principle—cook once, eat twice (or three times). If you make two big meals on a Sunday afternoon, you can actually feed yourself and your family for most of the week. Even if that means you fire up the grill and cook a bunch of salmon and chicken. You can turn that cooked protein into a variety of salads, meals, and soups during the week.

If you prepare a bit, when you get home on a weekday from work and the hungries are tempting you to call for take out—you'll have a solution that's healthier and less expensive!

Gluten-Free, Carolina-Style Barbecue Sauce

Cris often makes homemade sauces to enhance our meals. You can, too, and it'll help you make cooking and leftovers even more versatile. This sauce is an antidote to the processed, yucky, "heavy", ketchup-style sauces at the supermarket.

Ingredients:

1 cup white wine vinegar

1 cup apple cider vinegar

2 tablespoons brown sugar

1 teaspoon cayenne

1 tablespoon of your favorite pepper sauce (we use some of the hotter, habanero sauces)

2 teaspoons salt

1 teaspoon ground pepper

1 tablespoon smoked paprika

4 tablespoons tomato paste

1. Place all ingredients in a jar and shake.
2. Let it sit in the refrigerator for a day or two before using.

If refrigerated, it will last for 7–10 days.

Note: This sauce is very similar to some of the Carolina barbecue sauce recipes found online. It's great on top of shredded pork or grilled chicken. It can be also used as a marinade for other barbecued meats.

Watermelon-Infused Gazpacho

I've always loved the chilled, summer soup called gazpacho. A few years ago, a restaurant served me a version with an out-of-this-world watermelon flavor. Here's my version:

Ingredients:

2 cups organic tomato juice

2 cups watermelon juice

4 cloves garlic, peeled and chopped

1 tablespoon chopped fresh jalapeño

¼ cup balsamic vinegar

¼ cup extra-virgin olive oil

4 medium-sized ripe tomatoes, chopped

2 cucumbers, peeled, seeded and chopped

1 medium sweet onion (candy, Texas sweet, or Vidalia)

1 red bell pepper, cored, seeded, and chopped

Sea salt, to taste

NOTE: Fresh-juiced tomato and watermelon is best. Whole watermelon fruit (not rind) will liquefy in most blenders if you don't have a juicer available. Bottled tomato juice is your best substitute.

1. Mix together juices, garlic, jalapeño, onion, vinegar, oil, and sea salt in the blender or food processor. Blend until smooth.
2. Mix remaining ingredients together in a bowl. If you like a less chunky soup, run these ingredients through blender or food processor until slightly chunky.

I recommend making both parts of this recipe ahead at least four hours to let flavors combine. Vegetables can be stored separate from broth so they stay crisp.

Optional garnishes: finely diced fresh avocado, small spoonful of sour cream, or plain Greek yogurt

Dessert

Sugar and pain-relieving choices

Sugar is dessert and dessert is sugar, right? Most of us who love dessert (count me in on that … remember the pie story!), know that sugar is a big part of this desire.

There's a pretty significant dark side to sugar, though, and if you're going to eat dessert, you need to be aware of this information. It's your call what to do with it, especially because I'm suggesting a *lot* of changes in your food choices. You definitely want to take this pain-relieving process step by step and not overcommit to changes you'll find hard to maintain.

Bottom line, know this: Sugar can damage your body. Just as you're starting to relieve your pain, you wouldn't want to feed and reinforce it.

Here are some facts to consider about how sugar links to pain. I hope you'll use this information to help you decide your next steps.

- Sugar can interfere with absorption of magnesium. Magnesium relaxes muscle and can help relieve pain levels.
- Sugar can cause arthritis, which causes a great deal of pain for many people.
- Sugar can contribute to osteoporosis. Strong bones play a big part in holistic pain relief.

- Sugar can change the structure of collagen—a significant component in connective tissue. Compromised connective tissue can increase muscle and other types of pain.
- Sugar can increase the body's fluid retention. Fluid is a function of inflammation, and connects to pain[19].

Maybe you're thinking that switching artificial sweeteners for sugar is your solution. Sorry to burst your bubble, but it isn't going to help your pain levels. Aspartame, a common artificial sweetener, is strongly linked to migraines. Did you know that in 2010 *Clinical and Experimental Rheumatology* published findings that also linked aspartame to fibromyalgia pain and fatigue?

For me, the question of artificial sweeteners goes back to great-grandmother foods. How would I explain aspartame (NutraSweet®), saccharin (Sweet N Low®), sucralose (Splenda®) or any other artificial sweetener to her? Would she automatically know what it was, like we do?

Here's another thing I'd like you to think about regarding sugar. Sugar causes abnormal cell growth. Most people would rightly link this to concerns about cancer, but that's another book. What I want to point out here is that many people with arthritis have a condition called nodules. Nodules are little lumps of tissue that grow near joints and can cause pain and discomfort. If nodules are a result of abnormal cell growth, is it possible that eliminating sugar would start to shrink them? Would sugar abstinence prevent the growth of more nodules? I'm not a scientist or a medical professional, but if I were a person living with nodules and the associated pain, I'd definitely try to give up sugar. Remember, inflammation and pain

[19] Suicide by Sugar: A Startling Look at Our #1 National Addiction. Nancy Appleton, PhD and G. N. Jacobs, 2009.

are bio-individual. Even if your doctor has never seen anyone with this kind of connection between a particular food and pain, that doesn't mean the connection isn't real for you in your body.

Practical Strategy

The biggest pitfall related to sugar is how addictive it can be. The craving for sugar can pop out of nowhere and overwhelm you sometimes, right? So, what can you do to help minimize or eliminate those cravings?

Sugar cravings are your body asking for energy. Are you giving yourself a chance to gain energy in a natural way? How's your sleep, for example? If you can improve the quality and quantity of your sleep, you can often reduce the need for artificially created energy from sugar. (Read on for some ideas about sleep.) If you can add some exercise to your day or week, you can also gain energy from increasing your activity level. We'll cover that more in later chapters as well, because I know exercise feels like an extra challenge when you're living with chronic pain.

- Are you hungry for calories or nutrition? When you start thinking about reducing chemicals and shifting to whole foods, you'll find that your body is receiving the nutrition it craves. Our bodies have a natural mechanism that encourages us to fulfill our nutritional needs. If you focus on fantastic fueling foods, you'll likely find that your nutritional needs are met long before the sugar cravings start.
- Reduce processed foods, especially simple carbohydrates. Simple carbs are the white flour and white sugar-based foods, so reducing them breaks the craving cycle! It may be hard for the first few days, but it's absolutely worth it in the long run.

- Balance protein and healthy fats to stabilize blood sugar. When you're craving sweets and responding to cravings, your blood sugar jumps all over the place. Protein and healthy fats will mellow those jumps and provide you with more consistent energy throughout your day. Remember that omega 3 healthy fats are anti-inflammatory, too.
- Don't forget to keep hydrated; that can make a huge difference in both sugar cravings and pain levels.
- How much Vitamin L is in your life? Vitamin L is the *love* in your life. Have you given some hugs today? When I'm in need of Vitamin L, I reach out and hug my family, friends and clients. Every hug you give is a hug you get. Sometimes our cravings for sweets in food are really cravings for some sweetness in our lives. Take some time with a journal, therapist, or supportive friend to investigate this for you. You may find that increasing Vitamin L decreases your need for sugar.

Blueberry Rhubarb Crisp

I love to make pie, but when the inevitable time crunches strike, I make a healthy fruit crisp instead. As a gluten-free person now, a few things need to change in my go-to fruit crisp recipe. I've tried a few different alternatives, which led me to the one I'm going to share with you. It's my favorite and super delicious!

As a kid, my dad grew rhubarb and the plant would get absolutely huge. We had rhubarb all the time, and by the time I was a teenager I never wanted to taste it again. Confession: I haven't been a teenager in a *long* time, and enough years have passed for me to like rhubarb again. In fact, I actually asked a client who's a gardener for a rhubarb root a few years ago. I'm harvesting and enjoying my own rhubarb now!

Of course, this recipe does include sweetness, but the sweet taste is gentle and the ingredients don't include refined white sugar. Coconut sugar is great to try if you haven't already. It won't raise blood sugar the way refined sugar does, and you can use it as a one-to-one substitution. You can also reduce the quantity if you prefer a more tart flavor.

Ingredients:

1 cup rolled gluten-free oats

½ cup all purpose gluten-free flour

½ teaspoon sea salt

1 teaspoon ground cinnamon

¼ cup butter, melted

4 tablespoons maple syrup

1 tablespoon tapioca

¼ cup coconut sugar

¼ cup unsweetened applesauce

2 teaspoons vanilla extract

5 stalks rhubarb, washed with leaf removed, chopped

2 cups blueberries (organic, fresh or frozen)

1. Preheat oven to 350°F.
2. Mix gluten-free oats, gluten-free flour, salt, and cinnamon together in a bowl. Add butter and maple syrup. Mix well and set aside.
3. In a small bowl combine fruits, tapioca, coconut sugar, applesauce, and vanilla. Put in a lightly oiled 8 × 8 baking dish.

4. Spoon the oat mixture evenly on top of the fruit.
5. Cover and bake 40 to 45 minutes. Uncover and bake 10 minutes more to crisp the topping.

Events Away From Home

Now that we've covered the various times you're likely to be cooking at home, we should face the facts. It's unrealistic to think you'll be cooking at home 100% of the time. You'll have many opportunities to eat at restaurants, parties and other events, and it's important to plan some strategies to stay in the pain-relieving zone.

Restaurant Realities

I've learned to scope out restaurant websites and menus. Many menus are posted online now, so you can generally find something gluten-free almost anywhere you'd want to dine. You're lucky to be making these changes at a time when awareness has increased, because restaurant servers, chefs, and owners are really stepping up to the gluten-free plate.

Sometimes eating companions like certain places and may not be interested in changing their preferred dining destinations. With a little research first, it's possible to make anti-inflammatory and gluten-free restaurant meal choices. You'll want to do some up-front learning about what types of ingredients are "trouble spots." Then you may need to ask a few more questions when you're ordering, but ultimately eating out in a pain-relieving way *is* possible.

Cris and I love to eat out at great restaurants, but since going gluten-free for holistic pain relief, I've found it more challenging to be comfortable with our restaurant choices. I love the websites Yelp.com and UrbanSpoon.com for scoping out restaurants with gluten-free options. Both sites allow you to pick the "Gluten-Free Friendly" Feature to narrow your search based on user comments. Although these sites also have smart phone apps, unfortunately they aren't as helpful for gluten-free suggestions. In that case, I use my smartphone's browser to get into the site.

Once you reach the restaurant (if you can't research online in advance), ask for GF menus at the hostess stand. Take a minute to review the choices and be sure it suits you before you sit down and commit to stay at that restaurant. It's best to let your server know right away about your special diet needs. Getting help is key to making the experience positive for everyone involved—especially you. It's better to ask questions before ordering than to have to send something back or get gluten in your system. In addition to taking care of and pleasing yourself, you also make it easier on your server as well as your dining companions when you know your needs and order accordingly.

Pick one or two menu items that seem to be essentially gluten free, and ask your server to verify with the chef. Be familiar with typical gluten-containing ingredients in sauces and marinades—like soy sauce or Worcestershire sauce. Many restaurants are quite familiar with which ingredients contain wheat and gluten. I've even had some kitchen staff bring out their questionable ingredients so I could help them answer my own question! It's tempting to doubt that the restaurant staff cares about customer service, but you'll do yourself a favor to trust that this is *exactly* what's important to them.

Get familiar with possible sources of cross-contamination. For example, ask if french fries are breaded or battered. Even if they aren't, they may be fried in the same oil as other items that are breaded. You need to ask both questions—are they

GF, and are they prepared in a GF fryer (or other applicable environment)?

You may want to use the "pick my battles" strategy of GF ordering. If you've asked a ton of questions about the entrée, perhaps just ask for oil and vinegar in the bottle instead of also asking about which dressings are GF. When in doubt, you can always ask for a completely plain protein, but be sure to request "dry," with absolutely no seasoning at all. This is hard for chefs to do because they want to make food tasty—but it is critical to your health, so if you are taking your pain-relief food choices seriously, you need to insist. You can also ask for plain steamed vegetables—again, ask for no seasonings and a lemon slice or two on the side. Lemon can add a nice flavor to chicken, fish, or vegetables, and since you add it yourself, you know it's gluten free.

Practical Strategy

Going out for meals can sometimes be the most nerve-wracking part of being gluten free. There are so many people in a restaurant kitchen, and not all of them will be attentive to your particular needs. But know this—more people than ever are asking for specific dietary modifications when they order. Most restaurants will have encountered a gluten-free request before, so you're not going to surprise them as much as you think.

Most importantly, take this to heart: You are 100% worthy of the customer service it takes to keep you gluten free for pain-relief dining. Keep that in mind, and ask kindly and calmly for what you need; then tip your server generously as gratitude.

Party Healthy

I find it more challenging to stay anti-inflammatory at a party than in a restaurant. This is mainly because of the emotions and interpersonal relationships involved. The host or hostess has gone to a lot of trouble to create a wonderful menu. What happens when I have to decline an item—or a few items? Sometimes I worry I'll be hurting their feelings, but honestly, if I don't decline that item it's going to hurt me. In the end, it's worth a little bit of discomfort to protect my health and my body from inflammation and pain.

I've learned a few strategies that I believe may help you. For example, whenever possible, offer to bring a dish to a party. This way you know you'll always have something safe to eat. If the menu is a buffet or open house format, sometimes it's best to eat something at home before you go to the party. Just recently I had my protein at home and snacked on the fresh fruit and vegetables at an open house. I never felt like I was out of place, I didn't ingest anything harmful to my system, and I wasn't hungry or tempted. Hunger in a party or restaurant setting can do you in. It's hard to make anti-inflammatory choices when your stomach is growling and you feel light-headed. I often put a couple of safe snacks in my bag. This way I have a fall back plan if the party food isn't going to be fun for me later.

Alcohol

As with all the specifics relating to gluten, the topic of which alcohols and brands are appropriate for pain-relieving food choices is too large to cover here. My best advice is to visit the websites for the manufacturers of your favorite adult beverages. Look in the FAQ section of each site, and you'll often find allergy-related information.

Gluten-free choices are out there. However, with some other pain-related conditions like migraine, the connection between alcohol and pain is completely individual. You may find that you can drink one type of red wine, but not another. In some cases, it's not the alcohol that's the issue but the type of grape, the fermentation process, and the additives. Since it's also full of sugar and empty calories, you'll need to assess how important alcohol is to your lifestyle, relative to the importance of taking holistic steps to relieve your pain. It's all about balance and making the best choices for your bio-individual needs, and no one else can make those decisions for you.

Making Pain-Relieving Food Choices When You Travel

Like many of us, you may use routine and discipline as key elements in your effort to stay healthy; but when you take a trip, all of your usual routines can go out the window. Discipline is easy when you have control of your environment, but travel generally puts you out of control and into unknown territory.

What can you do to stay as healthy as possible when you are away from home? Here are seven simple tips to incorporate on your trips:

1. Try not to use the trip as one giant "treat meal."

   I remember when a weekend trip was my opportunity to "cheat" for 2–3 days. I also remember when it was easy to recover from that trip. It's not so easy now, in my late 40s. There's a lot to be said for keeping a degree of discipline while you travel. How much discipline is up to you, but it can make you feel more at home in unfamiliar places.

2. In airports, find a quiet(er) place to eat. Make the experience as much like a regular meal as possible.

   Airports are full of chaos, constant noise, and movement. Eating in this type of environment can often make us eat extremely quickly, which results in overeating or digestive issues. Since neither of those things are comfortable during a trip, try to find a somewhat peaceful spot for your meal. Get your food to go, and walk all the way to the end of the concourse. You'll get some additional space, plus a few extra steps of exercise. Find the least busy restaurant (which often is the one with healthier choices) and eat there. Sit at a table as far away from the edge of foot traffic as possible. Remember to breathe and fully chew your food.

3. Make water your main beverage for air/car/train travel.

   Plain bottled water has so many benefits for our bodies. No calories, no sodium, and pure hydration. It supports healthy digestion and fills us up so we snack less. Stick to water during your travel days instead of soda, alcohol, or juice.

4. Eat plenty of fruits and vegetables.

   Many fast food stops now offer fruits and vegetables on their menus or at the counter. Pick up a banana or an apple in the airport terminal to replace the snacks on the plane; or, choose a salad with limited cheese, fried toppings, and dressing. Focus on the vegetables in the salad instead.

5. Think about and plan ahead for your entire day's meals.

   Whether you're traveling or have reached your destination, make your meal and snack choices mindfully. If breakfast is the only meal where you'll be able to choose the source, choose healthier options for breakfast. If every meal choice is up to you, enjoy some healthy dining venues in your travel location.

6. Use online and smart phone apps that lead you to healthier choices.

When I was a kid, we always took a AAA guidebook on our vacations. We used the book to find things to do, along with restaurant choices. It's pretty wonderful when you consider how far we've come from that static, outdated information. Nowadays there are many valuable online resources you can use to find healthy, quality food choices on the road. In airports, I like the GateGuru app. In a new city, I use the UrbanSpoon and Yelp apps and websites when choosing restaurants. The reviews from real people are incredibly helpful.

7. Pack one small bar of decadent dark chocolate (unless it's a migraine trigger for you) and use it as your sweet treats for the entire trip!

   As I've said, sweets are the ongoing temptation for me. Before I travel, I now pack a bar of dark chocolate in my bag. After choosing to skip all the overly-indulgent sweets during the day, I will often treat myself to just one square of that dark chocolate at the end of the day. I find it helps me when I aim for "healthier" instead of "perfect" while traveling.

Rethinking Your Kitchen

Once you've decided to go gluten free, you can either reorganize or clean out your kitchen. There are lots of ways to accomplish this without inconveniencing other members of your household. You might decide to set aside certain cabinets or shelves for GF products, or you can mark everything that's GF and mix it all in together. Whatever seems easiest is best.

Of course, if you're cleaning out altogether then find friends, charities, or other folks who'd be interested in your gluten-containing foods. You can also donate foods you're giving up to a local food kitchen or possibly to your children's school for snacks.

Cross-contamination

When making a change to gluten-free foods, you'll want to understand cross-contamination. Food containing gluten can lurk in a lot of places in your kitchen—dishes and silverware that aren't completely clean is one place. Your countertop, cutting boards, and toaster also tend to hold onto crumbs. No matter who's going gluten-free, it's worth taking some time for a thorough cleaning.

Another place gluten-related crumbs will lurk is your sponges or on other cleaning cloths. Did you know you can throw sponges in the dishwasher? It's a great way to get them thoroughly clean, free of both gluten and germs.

Other cross-contamination sources to be aware of are jars of nut butter, mayonnaise, mustard, etc. Let's say one of the kids uses a knife to spread nut butter on his sandwich. His bread has gluten in it, and getting enough nut butter on the slice takes two or three dips into the jar. That knife just put gluten into your nut butter. It may be a pretty small amount, but multiply that by two slices of gluten-full toast each day, and there's a bunch of gluten in that jar.

I recommend labeling the jars you'd like to remain gluten-free. You can use old-fashioned canning labels, or even a labeler. I also found the loveliest labels and tags from a mom with celiac disease at http://www.glutenfreelabels.com.

Cookware

There's mounting evidence that chemicals used in non-stick cookware, perfluorooctanoic acid (PFOA) and perfluorooctane sulfonate (PFOS), may contribute to the alteration of natural hormones in our bodies that influence inflammation, cartilage repair, and systems of the body associated with arthritis. Featured in the *American Journal of Epidemiology*, Dr. Kim Innes of the School of Medicine at West Virginia University studied the connection between PFOA, PFOS (which are in most non-stick cookware and Teflon) and arthritis. The study collected data from 50,000 adults living in an area where they were exposed to PFOA and PFOS in the air as well as drinking water. It didn't even cover the topic of what type of cookware they used because the environmental exposure was so high.

Dr. Innes' study found that the people with the highest blood levels of PFOA were 40% more likely to develop arthritis, while adjusting for other factors such as age, weight, and gender. The connection between PFOA and arthritis was *strongest* in people who were younger and not obese. Since age and obesity are two known risk factors for osteoarthritis, that finding strengthens the apparent link, the researchers note.

These are your choices for cookware materials:

Potentially pain-relieving:

- Copper
- Stainless steel
- Cast iron
- Enameled cast iron
- Carbon steel
- Enamel on steel
- Green pan (a ceramic-based non-stick material)

Concerning—medically or potentially contributing to pain:

- Non-stick (correlations with pain and arthritis)
- Aluminum (possible correlation between aluminum and Alzheimer's disease)
- Anodized aluminum (possible correlation between aluminum and Alzheimer's disease)

After considering the above materials, I recommend you use stainless steel, which is what I use at home. You may ask, what's the difference between one stainless steel set and another? The primary difference will be the thickness of the steel and whether or not it's "multiclad/tri-ply" or aluminum layered in the stainless steel (both on the bottom and sides of the pot/pan). This is important since stainless steel is not a good conductor of heat.

You may be concerned about giving up the ease of cleaning a non-stick pot. I can honestly say that it's much less of an issue in our kitchen than I anticipated. If you can't clean something soon after eating, you'll need to fill it with hot water and some dishwashing detergent, then let it soak. In most cases, a good stainless surface isn't any more difficult to clean than non-stick coating.

Part Three

The Human Aspects of Holistic Pain Relief

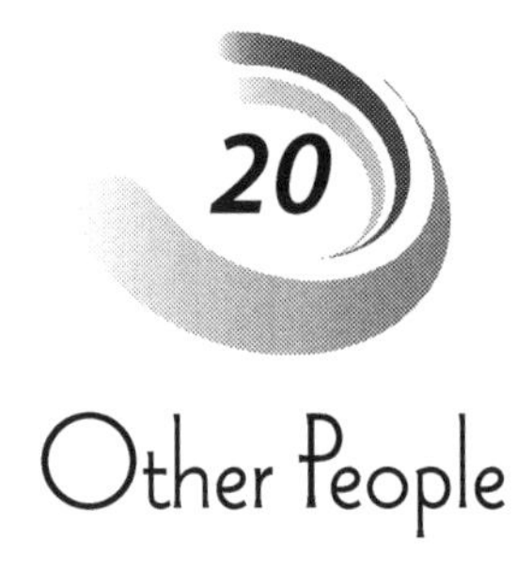

Other People

When I was first making some of these pain-relieving choices, it didn't really affect the other people in my life. I could switch my breakfasts easily, since I'm generally on my own for that meal. When my choices started to impact our family meals, however, I started to get a little nervous about how the changes would go over. Would Cris and the family think I was being a pain?

Of course, when I reached out and asked for help, I found that my family *wanted* me to feel better, and they've been willing to adjust their own lives to support me.

Whatever your reason for making pain-relieving choices, I encourage you to believe you're *100% worth* the care and attention it'll take to make the change. Healing your body and relieving your pain are incredibly important to your whole life. You *are* deserving of all the tools to make that possible!

Talking to Loved Ones (Especially Partners) About Going Gluten Free

When you live with someone else, you may worry that it'll be hard to go gluten free. Maybe they don't have the same health concerns or motivations you do, and you're concerned that they'll object even though they love you. Maybe they're the primary chef in the household, and you're not sure how much this change will affect them. No matter what the reason for your desire to change, it's always best to talk it over with your household family members. When you're ready to talk the GF change over with family, you may want to start with your spouse or partner. Once you've gained their support, you can work together on the best way to discuss this with the whole family.

First, find a time when you and your loved one are relaxed and can focus on each other for 15–20 minutes; maybe over a meal, or after the kids have gone to bed. Maybe you have a few moments in the car on the way to an event. You know your life. Choose this moment wisely, but don't agonize about it. Your goal is to start the conversation, not to do all the convincing at once. There are a lot of layers to this decision, and it may take a few different discussions to cover them all. Remember that your family loves you and wants you to be as pain-free as possible. That's your goal and they can't help but want to support you, because it'll ultimately benefit them, too.

Connecting With Others Helps Minimize Pain

During the times of chronic pain in my life, I've developed what I now call a "healing team." These are people in my life, both professionals and friends, who help me understand, heal, and manage my pain levels.

Lets start with the friends on your healing team. Chances are good that you know the people in your life who give you positive energy, and those who don't. One of my old bosses calls them the "sappers" and the "zappers". Sappers take your energy and don't give back. Zappers are the people who zap you with good energy, so you leave that connection with something positive.

Choose the zappers in your life for maximum pain-relieving support. Hang out with *those* friends—especially the friends you laugh with. Instead of just wishing you spent more time with friends, make a plan to see friends a certain number of times each month. Then, reach out to them and see what comes together. You can meet at a café, go for a walk, or just invite them to your home for a cup of tea. Getting online can help sometimes, too.

When I was first diagnosed with inflammatory autoimmune arthritis, I only knew a few people like me locally. I decided to start following people on Twitter who also mentioned arthritis in their profiles. Within a few weeks, I had a group of "peeps" who were feeling what I was feeling. Even though we couldn't meet for tea, I could shout out to the Twitterverse about my aches and pains and receive support.

Worth noting: too much of a good thing can be counterproductive. Did you know that there's a connection between how you feel about yourself and the time you spend on Facebook[20]? Sure, we make positive connections with new and old friends, and some folks have beautiful images and good ideas in their posts; but Facebook can also be a vehicle for comparison, and that's not always healthy.

Maybe you've heard the Teddy Roosevelt quote, "Comparison is the thief of joy." It's one of my favorite reminders to step away from the digital world sometimes.

In terms of healing professionals, I encourage you to ask trusted family, friends, and colleagues for recommendations. Sometimes you'll meet someone new and hear about strategies they use to manage their own health. Don't hesitate to ask questions and be open to learning new ideas for your own journey. When I get a new recommendation or idea for a treatment option, I often take a moment of quiet and

[20] http://bits.blogs.nytimes.com/2014/05/12/study-finds-being-ignored-on-facebook-leads-to-a-lower-self-esteem/?_php=true&_type=blogs&_r=0

ask myself, *Is this idea right for me right now?* When it feels intuitively right, I'll do some research and find the right professional. When a professional's name drops in your lap, often that's an inspiration worth follow up.

If a new treatment possibility doesn't feel right, simply put it into your "someday" category. The idea may come around again, perhaps at a time that's more logical for you.

You may not want to try all the holistic pain relief strategies you hear about all at once anyway, since it can be overwhelming. Give yourself permission to take one step at a time. Listen to your body's intuitive wisdom. What feels right?

Your Takeaway:

- Enjoy daily laughter.
- Ask supportive friends and family for help.
- Say no to events or environments that feel wrong.

But You Don't Look Sick

Many times people who live with chronic pain look just like everyone else in the family photo. But you know better, don't you? I know I do. No matter how normal you look today, people around you can't always understand how much more effort it takes to look like you're well. Friends and colleagues forget you have chronic pain, simply because you look pretty and not sickly.

When I was first diagnosed with arthritis, my social media pals introduced me to ButYouDontLookSick.com. The author, Christine Miserandino, had heard the comment about how "normal" she looked many times despite the chronic illness and pain she experienced daily. Christine developed a way of explaining her daily experience called "The Spoon Theory." (http://www.butyoudontlooksick.com/wpress/articles/written-by-christine/the-spoon-theory/) It's now been translated into multiple languages and spawned the "spoonie" movement. I hope these resources help you explain what life's like with chronic pain to others.

People Who Sabotage

Are there people you love who don't understand the choices you make? You're not alone! Those people may want you to feel better; they may even feel sad that you hurt a lot, but they don't always support you quite the way you'd like them to. What then?

I recently saw this exchange between a mother and daughter on Facebook. It was so indicative of this loving sabotage situation that I actually saved it to share with you:

Mother: You are going to have to endure a B-I-G cheat on Friday.

Daughter: Nope. I will bring myself stuff I can eat if I need. LOL

Mother: Oh I wish you wouldn't do that. Surely you can allow yourself to enjoy what I'm offering. You'll live through it.

This daughter didn't respond back to her mother. Would it have been hard for you to respond, too? I'm sure she didn't want to hurt her mother's feelings. I also imagine that the mother may not have realized how she might have hurt her daughter's feelings.

At what point is any particular food, no matter the love it was prepared with, worth additional (or any) pain the next day? Would the mother have asked a recovering addict to have a beer, just because she'd brewed it that day at home? Of course not.

These sabotaging people *do* love you; they just don't understand what living with chronic pain is like. I'm not suggesting you yell and scream at people who try to sabotage your holistic pain relief efforts, but I do encourage you to gracefully stand firm in what you know helps you.

You may want to develop a standard answer that helps in most situations. For example, you might say:

"I know how much you love me, and I appreciate that you want to give me this food tonight. I love you too. But I'm working hard to feel better, so we can spend more time together. For me, this means avoiding foods that increase my pain. The less pain I feel, the more energy I have, and I hope that means we can enjoy life together more! Would you please support me in this?"

You might go simple and direct instead:

"Thanks for your offer of _________ [fill in the food]. I know it's always been one of my favorites, but I will pay too big of a price in pain tomorrow. I'd love to share it with _________ [insert family or friend's name here] instead."

I know you'll find your own words. Remember you're not alone. Lots of people living with chronic pain run into this exact situation. So, reach out to your network and see what ideas they've tried as well.

Self-Care

All the food-related changes you'll make as you begin your holistic pain relief process will be enhanced when you're ready to take some steps towards self-care. Both paths are a journey towards acknowledging your self-worth. Sometimes we reach a bend in the road, or a few bigger pebbles, but I encourage you to consider these ideas. You'll find that adding them step-by-step into your life will bring you positive change.

How You Sleep is How You Do Everything

One of my mentors repeats this quote often. "How you do anything is how you do everything." Thinking of holistic pain relief, I like to say, "How you *sleep* is how you do everything."

What does this really mean? To me, it means if you sleep well, you spend the day feeling well. If you don't sleep consistently or deeply, it's hard to be consistent about anything you do during the day. If it hurts to sleep, chances are you are hurting during the day, too.

Does chronic pain make sleep more difficult? Or does difficulty sleeping make chronic pain worse? Honestly, I don't think it matters *which* is true. Both situations make your life more difficult if you can't find a way to improve them.

You and I both know that friends and family don't always understand what it's like to live with chronic pain. Chances are they may not understand what it's like to have chronically disturbed sleep, either. Jill Knapp writes in The Huffington

Post: "Most likely, a person in chronic pain isn't sleeping as well as they should. This could be because they are in too much pain to fall asleep, or to stay asleep, or they are having anxiety over the fear of dealing with pain for the rest of their life."

So, what're you, a person living with chronic pain, to do?

One thing you *don't* want to do is drink more caffeine. It's our society's go-to solution for the occasional sleepless night, but a 1997 study showed that patients with chronic back pain consume more than *twice* as much caffeine as patients without chronic back pain. In the same study, anecdotes suggested that using excess caffeine may also be associated with chronic back pain.

So, not only does caffeine potentially increase pain levels, but it can really mess with your ability to sleep. When I was still drinking a mug of coffee in the morning, I was taking a natural sleep aid supplement at night. When I quit the coffee, I no longer needed the sleep aid.

The good news is that there are some foods you can eat more of to get a better night's sleep. A 2012 study showed that the more varied your diet is, the better you'll sleep; so try new, healthy, whole foods and get plenty of variety throughout the day, week, and month. As tempting as it is to have the same breakfast or lunch every day, this is a *great* reason to switch it up regularly.

The study also shows that getting more lycopene, selenium, and vitamin C can improve sleep. The best sources of lycopene are grapefruit, tomatoes, papaya, and watermelon. There's a lot of selenium in shellfish, turkey, brazil nuts, and some types of fish. And broccoli and kale are two fantastic sources of vitamin C. These nutritious foods can each provide multiple benefits. How great is that?

Here's another interesting idea to consider—be sure to brush your teeth immediately after you wake. Why? Because arthritis has been linked to the bacteria gingivitis—it's actually been found in the *joints* of people diagnosed with inflammatory autoimmune arthritis.

7 Tips for a Better Massage When You Live with Chronic Pain

When you live with chronic pain, friends may suggest getting massage or bodywork to feel better. Maybe you've already had several massages over the years. In case you haven't noticed, sometimes a massage isn't a pleasant experience. It might hurt during the massage, or you might be uncomfortably sore for a few days afterward. Since I live with chronic pain like you, I've experienced this myself.

Here are my best suggestions for receiving massage as a positive experience. As a massage therapist, I always take these ideas into account when I see clients who live with chronic pain.

1. Less is more. Less pressure is better when you get on the table with chronic pain. This will be different than your friends who have short-term, situational pain. You don't need a deep tissue massage to relax, so simply ask for a relaxation or Swedish massage. In fact, if you're subconsciously bracing against deep massage pressure, the massage will be counterproductive. Relaxation massage can actually help chronic pain as much or even more than deep tissue massage.
2. It is especially helpful to find a therapist who specializes in massage for chronic pain, as they'll be the most understanding of your challenges. Look for a massage therapist who will work gently; who doesn't need to fix all your aches and pains in the first 60 minutes. Use this search

as a starting point (although you may want to narrow it down to your local area): http://www.amtamassage.org/findamassage/results.html?q=chronic+pain&l=&searchcat=famt

3. When you're looking for a new long-term massage therapist, ask what percentage of their clients have chronic pain. Massage designed to alleviate *chronic* pain is completely different than massage used for *acute* pain relief. Look for a therapist whose patients with chronic pain comprise at least 50% of their practice, and you'll be on the right track.
4. You might want to ask around to see if you can find a massage therapist who also lives with chronic pain. There's no directory that lists professionals by life experience, but sometimes friends and family will have a lead on the right therapist. When the person giving the massage has experienced their own chronic pain, they typically have a whole different understanding of your concerns.
5. Be willing to try different types of massage than what you may have received in the past. For example, one of the massage types I practice is called myofascial release (MFR). I'll explain more about it in the next section, as it's quite helpful for chronic pain. Physical and occupational therapists also get trained in MFR, so sometimes you can get it covered by insurance if your doctor writes a prescription.
6. Don't be afraid to ask for special accommodations during your massage. For example, if you struggle to turn from your belly to your back, ask to start on your back so the turning is easier. If heat on the table makes you feel looser, be sure to request it. On the other hand, if you're more uncomfortable with too much heat, don't be shy about requesting a cool table. These may seem like small details,

but trust me, no detail is too small if it means you get the help you need.

7. Choose a massage therapist whose office is relatively close to home. It sounds silly, but after you get relaxed you don't want a long drive that might make you feel tense again.

The bottom line is that a great massage starts with effective communication. This is even more important when you live with chronic pain. Be sure your therapist is open to requests, and remember that *you* are the most important person in that treatment room. Your therapist really does want you to be clear about what you need, so never worry about asking.

Myofascial Release: A Different Kind of Bodywork

About 10 years ago I received my first myofascial release (MFR) bodywork treatment. Since then I've spent over 140 hours in training to be a MFR therapist, and many hundreds more treating clients. I've also benefited greatly from the holistic approach of the MFR bodywork I've received. It's an effective method of treating chronic pain because it helps relieve existing pain while also offering an avenue to start resolving long-term causes and dysfunctions.

Ginevra Liptan, M.D. quotes a patient in her book *Figuring Out Fibromyalgia:* "Myofascial release works better than any pill to relieve my pain."

The type of MFR I practice, and what Dr. Liptan references in her book, is taught by John F. Barnes, P.T. While there are many therapists offering myofascial work, I believe the Barnes approach is far superior for most people. It's worth searching out someone trained in this particular approach. MFR uses gentle, hands-on pressure to engage the fascial system and restore health and balance throughout your body. This inherently safe process facilitates your body's natural ability to unwind, release subconscious holding patterns, and thus reintegrate the body, nervous system, and mind. The result is significant change that's measurable and functional.

Fascia is a type of tissue that creates a three-dimensional, whole-body system. It supports and protects every system—muscle, nerve, bone, joint, blood vessel, organ, and cell in the body. Imagine it as an intricately connected web that reaches from head to toe in each of us. This web is made up of fibers and a fluid ground substance. Myofascial restrictions are created when the fluid aspect of the fascia loses its gel-like properties as a result of injury, inflammation, surgery, stress, poor posture, and/or repetitive strain. Restrictions can create pressure up to 2000 lb. per square inch. That's like having two horses standing on one square inch of your body! Your body tries to accommodate these restrictions by adjusting posture, motion, and flexibility. Over time this causes pain, weakness, inflammation, or malfunction throughout the body, sometimes with symptoms that seem unrelated. MFR is a profound solution.

A variety of therapists can be trained in MFR—physical therapists, massage therapists, occupational therapists, and speech therapists. During your first MFR appointment, the therapist will evaluate your posture and then discuss treatment. Therapists may work throughout your body or on one specific area, depending on your treatment plan.

It's a different type of treatment from the massages most commonly experience. MFR using the Barnes approach will include long, slow, sustained holds. The myofascial restriction is lightly stretched or lengthened, and this position is maintained for at least two minutes, often longer. This process is then repeated throughout the body based on the therapist's assessment and your experience on the table. Treatment is non-injurious, and helps to heal mind, body, and spirit.

Check out a visual exploration of fascia here:

http://youtu.be/01jdrGrp4Fo.

Integrating Movement Into Your Day

Many people ask me what causes the pain they're experiencing. Sometimes we can point to a specific event, but that's fairly rare. Usually both acute and chronic pains have cumulative factors resulting from actions continued over long periods of time. So, I've developed a theory: there are just two causes for pain. The first cause is movement, and the second is lack of movement.

It sounds a bit cavalier, but after thousands of client appointments I believe it's a solid theory. Of course, every person and situation is individual, so these ideas are still generalizations and experiences may vary.

When the cause of pain is movement, the first type of pain comes from moving in a long-term, repetitive, dysfunctional way. An example of this might be sitting with poor posture for many years.

If the cause of pain seems to be simple, like a sneeze resulting in extreme pain, that's actually more likely to be caused by a long-term, untreated dysfunction. You've pushed the dysfunction to the limit of what it can withstand without adequate treatment, and it becomes painful.

Another cause of pain related to movement is overdoing a short-term movement where your muscles aren't accustomed to being used in that way. Examples would be shoveling snow, gardening in the spring, or playing a new sport.

A far more destructive chronic pain is due to lack of movement. Does your whole body feel incredibly stiff upon waking, and then feel better an hour later? Although you may have arthritis that explains this, perhaps it's also caused by the stillness of your sleep positions. I am always amazed when people ask if my massage therapy work makes me tired at day's end. In fact, I've experienced the opposite—giving several hours of massage is *less* tiring than sitting at a desk for the same amount of time. This was true even when I was living at the height of my chronic pain.

Here's why movement helps chronic pain: It produces endorphins, which help enhance your mood; and encephalin, which minimizes pain. Movement lubricates joints, moves oxygen and nutrition throughout our bodies, and even helps the body to cleanse toxins. In my research I found an interesting project called "Take-A-Stand". This program is designed to help people stop sitting still all day. The results of adding just one hour of non-sitting time each day are amazing. The project has found that with one less hour of sitting per day, participants reported 50% less pain, and 38% reported reduced fatigue. This is clear evidence that movement is a critical part of how you can reduce chronic pain. This doesn't mean you have to start running marathons. In fact, you just need to find small ways to start integrating movement into your day.

Start by adding 5 minutes of stretching to every day—or even 10 minutes. It doesn't have to be all at once. You may want to start gently stretching your neck when you're at the computer or in the car at a stoplight. Try doing some gentle forward bends at your desk, on the floor, or in your bed.

Another part of us that gets extra tight when we sit a lot is our hips. Tight hips will cause dysfunction throughout your core, from lower back down to the knees. The best and simplest antidote to this tension is to sit cross-legged—what we used to call Indian-style. When you're on the couch watching TV, sit this way for a bit. Or, if you read before bed, do this while you read. The reason these two places can be ideal is that you'll want to spend at least five minutes each day in this position; you want to be in a quiet moment of your day.

If your hips are so tight that your knees don't reach the couch or the bed, you can solve this by taking a pillow or two and placing them under your knees for support. As you progress and your hips begin to stretch, you'll need the pillows less and less.

Your Takeaway:

- Get up and move at least once each hour during the day.
- Assess your old movement strategies.
- Try a new way to exercise.

Would You Run a Mile in a Pool?

The other day I said something that I still think is brilliant. "I may not ever run a marathon, but I think my whole life is the marathon. I have to pace myself and work hard at today's race, so I can make it to the end in the best shape possible."

Now, by "best shape" I didn't mean a certain dress size. I meant living in a healthy and active way choosing to live the way *you* want to instead of letting chronic pain dictate your limitations.

Having lived with pain for most of my adult life (which I confess is now a couple of decades or so), I've developed some chronic pain relief strategies. In my twenties and thirties one of my key strategies was getting regular exercise, but as my pain progressed, my old exercise habits didn't suit me anymore. They actually generated more pain instead of fostering relief.

During this time, my aunt kept telling me how much she loved her water exercise classes in the pool. My perception of those classes was that the attendance was exclusively ladies

70+ in years. I thought I'd feel out of place. Boy, was I ever wrong! There are women (and a few brave men) from many different decades of life, including some over 80 years old, and others in their 30s and 40s.

Since I started taking water exercise classes a few years ago, it's been a valuable, pain-relieving experience. I was recently reminded how much I love it, because as I hopped in the pool after several weeks away, I felt like I was *home.*

Now, exactly why is water exercise so helpful when you live with chronic pain? 90% of our body is buoyant in water, so joints experience less stress with movement. This can be helpful when you live with conditions such as arthritis and fibromyalgia. Because water offers hydrostatic pressure (a constant weight in all directions), you receive 12%–14% more resistance in a pool. Muscles are actually strengthened with every move you make. As my friend and fellow author, Janet Hartlove, says, it's like you're wearing full body shape-ware when you exercise!

You'll find there are many benefits to water exercise. You'll hear about the way it strengthens your muscles, but I also want to point out that it makes you more flexible. After 12+ years of working with massage clients, I've learned that you can't trade flexibility for strength. You need both!

Water exercise may also benefit your mental health. Maybe it's the reminders of my childhood summers in the pool, but I almost always feel happy in the water. When you bust a move in the pool, you're generating your body's own feel-good hormones.

Statistically, if you're living with chronic pain you're more likely to live with depression. Getting in the pool can help you combat those feelings, and you'll enjoy getting to know the other students. The social connections are beneficial for holistic pain relief as well.

Negativity Detox

You may think that detoxifying your body is the most important part of feeling better, and making changes that stop you from taking in foods your body finds toxic is important, to be sure; but have you ever thought about the way you *think* affecting your pain levels? I believe that having a negativity detox plan is absolutely critical to any holistic pain relief plan. This is all up to you, and not something you can pay someone to do for you. It's also my personal philosophy, so if it doesn't resonate with you, that's okay. It's especially important to keep in mind how you refer to and discuss your story of living with chronic pain. Here's what I mean: When I was first diagnosed with inflammatory autoimmune arthritis, I was immediately concerned about the type of language that is used to describe autoimmune disease. Autoimmunity is a condition where part of your immune system is overactive towards your body. Notice I said overactive—but typical medical language says that the immune system *attacks* the body. I decided soon after my diagnosis to *never* use that phrasing when I was talking about myself. It didn't seem productive, since my main goal was to find healing and pain relief, not *war* and *fighting*.

I'm not encouraging you to be dishonest about your pain or your diagnosis when someone asks, but instead to look for the most positive possible way to frame the situation.

For example, people ask me: How is it possible for you to do massage with autoimmune arthritis? My answer: I've never NOT done massage with arthritis, so it seems normal to me.

I believe this attitude helps me to keep pursuing a highly physical career, no matter my diagnosis.

When you feel limited on any given day, try to focus on what you *can* do instead of what you *can't.* Remember, every moment you're up and moving around is a privilege, because I'm sure you know people whose pain immobilizes them and makes them 100% dependent on others.

So ask yourself: "What do I *get* to do today?" instead of "What can't I do?"

Mindset and Holistic Pain Relief

Last year I attended a retreat about our mindset—the way we approach our lives, relationships, career, and success. It was an amazing event that I couldn't help but connect to holistic pain relief. What I learned is that mindset is the combination of three things: thoughts, beliefs, and actions.

How does that relate to living with chronic pain? Do you find yourself thinking about your discomfort and pain all the time? Or maybe you believe that the pain will never end. If you live with pain, you may find that you don't take action because you feel hopeless and miserable.

What would happen if you could make a decision to change your mindset today? You could:

- Think about pain relief solutions.
- Believe that small changes can add up to big gains.
- Take action to change your habits in ways that support pain relief.

Remember, I've been on both sides of this coin. I had my first experiences of chronic back pain in my twenties, without realizing it wasn't how all my friends felt. After finding help from chiropractic treatment, I felt pretty good for a few years.

Then the back pain returned with a vengeance in my early thirties. This time it was massage therapy that helped me manage and heal the pain.

With the autoimmune arthritis diagnosis in my forties, I had a much bigger mindset challenge because chronic illness felt so much scarier than back pain.

I've been in your shoes!

So, how do you change the way you're thinking about holistic pain relief? Well, being part of a pain-relief community is a good place to start. When you connect with like-minded individuals who are also focused on solutions instead of tied to the pain experience, you're supported and can feel more positive. You'll find that taking time to laugh and enjoy life will make a mindset difference. For example, choose an uplifting comedy instead of a heavy drama when you go to the movies. Spend time with friends who are positive thinkers (zappers). Listen to happy music instead of news in the car. Make time for the goodness in life!

All of these things combine to help you shift your belief system.

Simply put, beliefs are thoughts you think over and over and over again.

Take some time (maybe with a journal) to reflect on the thoughts you were taught as a child about your body's health. For example, did your parents or grandparents often say things like, "Everyone's body falls apart after 40"? Perhaps you've internalized this belief without even realizing it.

Or do you say things like, "I hate how my body has stopped working," or just simply, "I hate my body" many times every day? Reframing these beliefs can make a world of difference for you.

The next step is to look beyond your thoughts and beliefs to the action steps that relate to your mindset. I encourage you to dream about the life you'd like to create for yourself. Start a vision board or make a "mind movie" that will give you visual and emotional cues. Take some time to imagine and visualize what you'd like your life to be. Maybe capture that vision in your journal, as well, and keep revisiting your vision on a daily basis.

In the past, maybe you've decided to take action and chosen the top twenty things you need to change, then tried to change them all at once. From my personal experience, this is a recipe for frustration and maybe even disaster.

If you're contemplating the changes I've shared here in this book, please consider changing just one thing at a time. Determine which *one change* you'll start with, and then make a plan that helps you make that one change. Live with that change for a bit—days or even weeks; then consider adding another change into your life. Continue on until you find your pain has been relieved. Step-by-step adjustments give you a pace that both acknowledges and addresses the chronic pain in your life.

Be easy with yourself as you move forward.

Part Four

Are You Ready for a Fresh Start?

I love this quote from author and poet, Mark Nepo: "When my pockets are empty and I've dumped all I know, I often end up shrugging, admitting my ignorance of what to do. Humbly, it is then that the real work of love begins."

This may feel like a huge bundle of new information to take in because I've "dumped my pockets." You may indeed feel like the one shrugging and wondering what to do next. This is the part where we both must begin the real work of love.

I'm here for you. I encourage you to use the Japanese concept called *kaizen.* I like to translate *kaizen* as "baby steps." The first step is deciphering your bio-individual puzzle, and loving yourself enough to make changes.

Particularly when you live with chronic pain, it's important to incorporate changes in a way that works for you. Don't let me or anyone else tell you how it's going to work in your life and your body!

If you feel overwhelmed or would just like some extra support to implement these ideas, that's the perfect time to reach out to me. I am currently accepting private clients, and available to speak to your group, company, or organization about holistic pain relief. I'll also be developing online group programs in the future.

I offer my private clients a customized, tested process called, "Unlocking the Puzzle of Pain." It's more detailed than the "baby steps" offered here. Of course, it also includes our personal connection and the coaching work we'd do together.

To spend 30 minutes on the phone with me discussing whether this is your next step, simply schedule your Fresh Start Phone Call here:

www.confidentwellness.com/i-need-a-fresh-start-now/

While there, I hope you'll download the free PDF report, *17 Easy Ways to Start Minimizing Pain Today!* (www.confidentwellness.com/17ways/)

Please join our online communities and conversations so you can receive support and gentle encouragement. You'll find our community most welcoming. We are online at:

www.confidentwellness.com/blog-2/

www.facebook.com/confidentwellness

www.twitter.com/confidentlywell

This book represents my own *kaizen* experience. The way chronic pain is treated in this country breaks my heart. I've met so many people during my journey who don't have the solutions they need to feel better. The price of pain is too high and the puzzle of solving it is too complicated.

I hope that by touching your life through this book and ConfidentWellness.com, we can work together to transform the experience of living with chronic pain, for you and for the world.

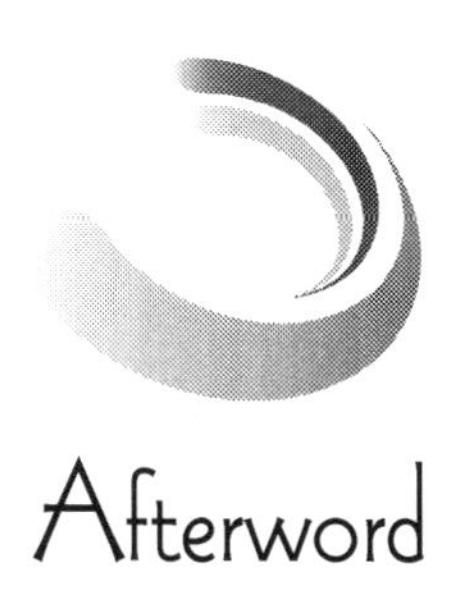

Afterword

Everyone's life is fluid, and mine is no exception. Even as this book was developing and moving towards publication, changes were happening in my health status. At the same time, it's the nature of writing to stop making revisions and publish. This means I haven't been able to capture the recent changes to my story here. I also hope you'll understand that adding more details of my life and health would have detracted from the central message of this book.

As I sort things through, you'll find me sharing and posting on my blog at ConfidentWellness.com as well as in a future book.

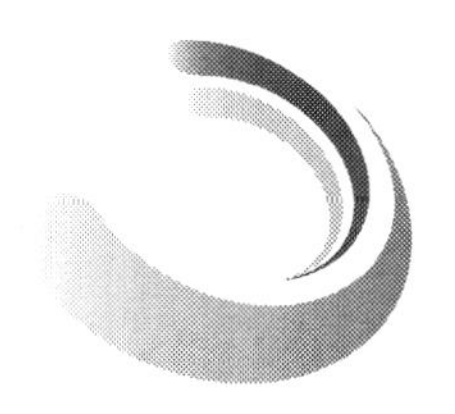

Acknowledgements

My massage and health coaching clients have been the light in each working day. I treasure our relationships, and look forward to many years to come.

Beth Kallman Werner, thank you for editing this book in a way that left my voice intact while improving every comma, sentence, and section. I trust you as a former colleague, friend, and now my editor.

Randy Graffa, thanks for evoking just the right feeling in this book's cover. Your design will make people click the button that begins them on a journey toward pain relief. It wouldn't have been the same without you.

Many thanks to each of the friends and colleagues who read early drafts of the book and offered feedback: Jen Viano, Liz Baak, Jane Coffman Swartz, RN, Judy Rizzo, Judy Flowers, Gina Harrison, Naomi Levine, Patricia Young, Dr. F. Gianmichael Salvato, Marilyn Hohenwarter, Beth Willson, Christine Minnich, Barbara Darnell, Carla Saylor, Kelly Scotti, Sandi Gordon, and Scott Harrison.

This book came to fruition during an online writing course led by Lindsey Smith and Joshua Rosenthal, founder of the Institute for Integrative Nutrition (IIN). Thank you for encouraging coaches and authors to rock the ripple effect of health and wellness.

I'm grateful for the learning and networking of Lancaster's Holistic Mastermind Group, led by Lori and Patrick Kirkham.

Jeannie Spiro and I first met as classmates at IIN, and her coaching helped start ConfidentWellness.com out on the right foot.

My experience with Fabienne Fredrickson and the Client Attraction Business School was unparalleled. I'm also especially thankful for the Accountability Buddies who supported me during that time: Stacy Rowan, Denise Lloyd, Terry Nicholetti, and Lisa Jackson.

In the book I talk about developing your own healing team. This book would never have seen the light of day without the care I receive from my healing team of health care professionals and practitioners of many types of healing.

I am blessed to be part of a large extended family of kids, grandkids, in-laws, former in-laws, nieces, nephews, aunts, uncles, and cousins. I love you all.

Aunt Judy, your listening ear, wisdom, and eggplant parmigiana are precious gifts. Thank you.

Dad, even though you aren't here to see the published book I know you're excited for me somewhere out there. I miss you.

Mom, your creative approach to life and writing inspired me to tell this story now and not later. You've been my chief encourager and confidante for longer than anyone else, and it means the world to me. Our book is next!

Cris, it's hard to imagine that first conversation about printer incompatibility has grown into twenty blissful years together. You've been my cheerleader from the very beginning, and it's never been more important than in the last few years. Thanks for taking this book from lowly MS Word to a beautiful, professional look. It's a joy to be your wife, life partner, business partner, and best friend. Here's to twenty more years!

About the Author

Barbara Searles, LMT, BCTMB, HHC, AADP is a nationally certified massage therapist and health coach. As the founder of ConfidentWellness.com, she's deeply passionate about coaching people living with chronic pain. Her strategies have been featured in *Health Monitor, Natural Awakenings,* and BlogTalkRadio. When she's not coaching, writing, or speaking, you'll find her relaxing with her family.

Made in the USA
Lexington, KY
23 April 2015